Contents

The National Collaborating Centre
for Chronic Conditions

Funded to produce guidelines for the NHS by NICE

ANAEMIA MANAGEMENT IN CHRONIC KIDNEY DISEASE

National clinical guideline for
management in adults and children

by

l College
hysicians

er medical standards

Mission statement

The Royal College of Physicians plays a leading role in the delivery of high quality patient care by setting standards of medical practice and promoting clinical excellence. We provide physicians in the United Kingdom and overseas with education, training and support throughout their careers. As an independent body representing over 20,000 Fellows and Members worldwide, we advise and work with government, the public, patients and other professions to improve health and healthcare.

The National Collaborating Centre for Chronic Conditions

The National Collaborating Centre for Chronic Conditions (NCC-CC) is a collaborative, multi-professional centre undertaking commissions to develop clinical guidance for the NHS. The NCC-CC was established in 2001. It is an independent body, housed within the Clinical Standards Department at the Royal College of Physicians of London. The NCC-CC is funded by the National Institute for Health and Clinical Excellence (NICE) to undertake commissions for national clinical guidelines on an annual rolling programme.

Citation for this document

National Collaborating Centre for Chronic Conditions. *Anaemia management in chronic kidney disease: national clinical guideline for management in adults and children.* London: Royal College of Physicians, 2006.

ISBN-13: 978-1-86016-293-0
ISBN-10: 1-86016-293-2

ROYAL COLLEGE OF PHYSICIANS
11 St Andrews Place, London NW1 4LE
www.rcplondon.ac.uk

Registered charity No 210508

Typeset by Dan-Set Graphics, Telford, Shropshire

Printed in Great Britain by The Lavenham Press Ltd, Suffolk

Members of the Guideline Development Group

Dr David Halpin *(Chair)*
Consultant Thoracic Physician, Royal Devon and Exeter NHS Foundation Trust

Dr Penny Ackland, Royal College of General Practitioners
General Practitioner, London

Dr Samir Agrawal, Royal College of Pathologists
Senior Lecturer, Queen Mary, University of London
Honorary Consultant in Haematology, Barts and The London NHS Trust

Ms Carol Anderson, Anaemia Nurse Specialist Association
Anaemia Nurse Specialist, East Kent Hospitals NHS Trust

Mr Robert Bradley, UK Renal Pharmacy Group
Pharmacist, Cardiff and Vale NHS Trust

Mr Robert Dunn, National Kidney Federation
Patient and Carer Representative, Devon

Dr Jonathan Evans, British Association for Paediatric Nephrology
Consultant Paediatrician, Nottingham City Hospital NHS Trust

Mrs Bernadette Ford, NCC-CC
Information Scientist

Dr Jane Fisher, NCC-CC
Project Manager (until July 2005)

Mr Rob Grant, NCC-CC
Senior Project Manager (from August 2005)

Ms Christine Howard, National Kidney Research Fund
Patient and Carer Representative, Devon

Ms Karen Jenkins, Royal College of Nursing
Anaemia Nurse Specialist, East Kent Hospitals NHS Trust

Dr Mick Kumwenda, British Renal Society
Consultant Renal Physician, Conwy and Denbighshire NHS Trust

Professor Alison MacLeod, Cochrane Renal Group
Consultant Nephrologist, Aberdeen Royal Infirmary
Professor of Medicine, University of Aberdeen

Dr Nyokabi Musila, NCC-CC
Health Services Research Fellow in Guideline Development (until February 2006)

Ms Debbie Nicholl, NCC-CC
Health Economist (until November 2005)

Dr Shelagh O'Riordan, British Geriatrics Society
Consultant Physician in Healthcare of Older People, East Kent Hospitals NHS Trust

Mrs Alison Richards, NCC-CC
Information Scientist

Ms Alison Roche, Anaemia Nurse Specialist Association
Nurse Consultant, King's College Hospital NHS Trust

Dr Paul Roderick, Faculty of Public Health
Senior Lecturer in Public Health, University of Southampton and Southampton University Hospitals NHS Trust

Dr Paul Stevens *(Clinical Adviser)*
Consultant Renal Physician, East Kent Hospitals NHS Trust

Dr Stephen Thomas, Royal College of Physicians
Consultant in Diabetes Medicine, Guy's and St Thomas' NHS Foundation Trust

Dr Eric Will, British Renal Society
Consultant Renal Physician, Leeds Teaching Hospitals NHS Trust

Ms Jane Alderdice was invited to contribute at a specific meeting as an expert representing the British Dietetic Association, but was not a full member of the GDG

Dr Luigi Gnudi acted as a deputy for Dr Stephen Thomas at a GDG meeting, representing the Royal College of Physicians

Acknowledgements

The Guideline Development Group is grateful to the following for their valuable contributions to the development of this guideline:

- Dr Bernard Higgins, Director, NCC-CC
- Ms Jane Ingham, Director of Clinical Standards, Royal College of Physicians of London
- Ms Ester Klaeijsen, Administrator, NCC-CC
- Mr Derek Lowe, Medical Statistician, Astraglobe Ltd
- Ms Jill Parnham, Manager, NCC-CC
- Mrs Susan Varney, Research Fellow, NCC-CC
- Colleagues working on the Health Technology Assessment of erythropoiesis-stimulating agents for cancer treatment-induced anaemia.

Preface

Chronic kidney disease (CKD) is not the most common cause of anaemia in the UK, but data from different sources suggest that nationally there are around 100,000 people with the combination of CKD and a low haemoglobin level. Anaemia in this context is important because it contributes significantly to the heavy symptom burden of CKD, and because it is potentially reversible with appropriate treatment, including erythropoietin. Erythropoietin is naturally produced by the kidneys and has been available in synthetic form for the treatment of anaemia of CKD since 1989, but it remains a fairly expensive product and its usage is not straightforward. Moreover, it will not necessarily be the only therapy required for optimal treatment. Against this background, the present guideline has been commissioned to address the appropriate management of anaemia of CKD for patients in the NHS.

The guideline has been produced using standard NICE methodology,[1] and is therefore explicitly evidence-linked. Following a comprehensive literature search and evaluation of research papers, a Guideline Development Group (GDG) comprising clinical experts and patient and carer representatives assessed the evidence and used it to produce a detailed set of recommendations. This was no easy task, but one which the GDG have carried out diligently, thoroughly and with patient good humour. They have been a pleasure to work with and all at the National Collaborating Centre for Chronic Conditions are grateful to them.

The guideline recommendations cover many aspects of anaemia management in CKD, but some deserve emphasis. The thresholds at which treatment should be considered receive deserved attention, as do target values for haemoglobin. The GDG were clear that treatment, including administration of erythropoiesis stimulating agents, should be considered for all ages when there is the prospect of improving physical function and quality of life. The importance of correctly managing iron status is emphasised as well as the role of erythropoiesis stimulating agents. The GDG also stressed the importance of agreeing a detailed plan with patients regarding all aspects of delivery of treatment.

There is no doubt that symptoms would be improved in many patients with CKD if anaemia were to be managed optimally. We hope and expect that this guideline will make a significant contribution to improving the lives of the patients who suffer from this debilitating condition.

Dr Bernard Higgins MD FRCP
Director, National Collaborating Centre for Chronic Conditions

DEVELOPMENT OF THE GUIDELINE

1 | Introduction

1.1 Definition of anaemia

Internationally anaemia is defined as a state in which the quality and/or quantity of circulating red blood cells are below normal. Blood haemoglobin (Hb) concentration serves as the key indicator for anaemia because it can be measured directly, has an international standard, and is not influenced by differences in technology. However, because haemoglobin values in healthy individuals within a population show a normal distribution, a certain number of healthy individuals will fall below a given cut-off point.

Conventionally anaemia is defined as a haemoglobin concentration lower than the established cut off defined by the World Health Organization (WHO),[2] and different biological groups have different cut-off haemoglobin values below which anaemia is said to be present. This cut-off figure ranges from 11 grams per decilitre (g/dl) for pregnant women and for children between 6 months and 5 years of age, to 12 g/dl for non-pregnant women, and to 13 g/dl for men (Table 1.1). No downward adjustment for the elderly is made for age. Although there is a theoretical basis for a fall in male haemoglobin levels with age, because of reduced testosterone production, this is clearly not the case for women. Furthermore there is accumulating evidence that anaemia reflects illness and is associated with adverse outcomes in the elderly.[3]

In the Cardiovascular Health Study 8.5% of participants were anaemic by WHO criteria. Those who were anaemic had a greater prevalence of associated comorbidity and significantly higher 11-year death rates than those without anaemia (57% and 39% respectively, p ≤0.001). The strongest correlates of anaemia were low body mass index, low activity level, fair or poor self-reported health, frailty, congestive heart failure, and stroke or transient ischemic attack. Anaemia was also associated with higher concentrations of creatinine, C-reactive protein, and fibrinogen, and lower levels of albumin and white blood cell count.[4]

Table 1.1 Haemoglobin cut offs to define anaemia in people living at sea level[2]	
Age or gender group	Haemoglobin below: (g/dl)
Children	
6 months to 5 years	11.0
5 to 11 years	11.5
12 to 14 years	12.0
Non-pregnant females >15 years	12.0
Men >15 years	13.0

In addition to gender, age, and pregnancy status, other factors influence the cut-off values for haemoglobin concentration. These include altitude, race, and whether the individual smokes. Although altitude is not a factor in patients in England, ethnicity may influence the cut-off values for haemoglobin concentration.

Data from the USA show that healthy people of African extraction of all age groups at all times, except during the perinatal period, have haemoglobin concentrations 0.5–1.0 g/dl below those of white people, a difference independent of iron-deficiency and socioeconomic factors.[5–9] Haemoglobin concentration increases in smokers because of the formation of carboxyhaemoglobin, which has no oxygen transport capacity.[10]

The US Centers for Disease Control and Prevention have developed a smoking-specific haemoglobin adjustment to define anaemia in smokers (Table 1.2) and suggest that these values should be subtracted from observed haemoglobin values.[11]

Table 1.2 Haemoglobin adjustment for smokers

Amount smoked	Haemoglobin adjustment (g/dl)
½–1 packs/day	0.3
1–2 packs/day	0.5
>2 packs/day	0.7
All smokers	0.3

1.2 Chronic kidney disease: definition and prevalence

The Renal National Service Framework[12,13] has adopted the US National Kidney Foundation Kidney Disease Outcomes Quality Initiative (NKF-KDOQI) classification of chronic kidney disease (CKD).[14] This classification divides CKD into five stages (Table 1.3) defined by evidence of kidney damage and level of renal function as measured by glomerular filtration rate (GFR).

Table 1.3 Stages of chronic kidney disease

Stage	GFR (ml/min/1.73m^2)	Description
1	>90	Normal or increased GFR, with other evidence of kidney damage
2	60–89	Slight decrease in GFR, with other evidence of kidney damage
3	30–59	Moderate decrease in GFR, with or without other evidence of kidney damage
4	15–29	Severe decrease in GFR, with or without other evidence of kidney damage
5	<15	Established renal failure

Stage 5 CKD may be described as established renal failure (also called end stage renal failure), and is CKD which has progressed so far that renal replacement therapy (regular dialysis treatment or kidney transplantation) will be required to maintain life. Established renal failure is an irreversible, long-term condition. A small number of people with established renal failure may choose conservative management only.

Conventionally, the total number of people receiving renal replacement therapy has been taken as a proxy measure for the prevalence of established renal failure. The National Service Framework (NSF) for renal services estimates that more than 27,000 people were receiving renal replacement therapy in England in 2001. Approximately one-half of these had a functioning transplant and the remainder were on dialysis. It is predicted that numbers will rise to around 45,000 over the next 10 years. However, the most recently published Renal Registry Report (2004) highlights that in the UK there were over 37,000 patients receiving renal replacement therapy during 2003, a prevalence of 632 per million population. Of these, 46% had a functioning transplant and the remainder were receiving dialysis treatment.[15]

Data from the third US National Health and Nutrition Examination Survey (NHANES III) suggests that overall 11% of the population have some degree of kidney disease: 3.3% of the population are in stage 1 CKD, 3.0% in stage 2 CKD, 4.3% in stage 3 CKD, 0.2% in stage 4 CKD and 0.2% in stage 5 CKD.[10] A similar population prevalence of stage 3–5 CKD has recently been described for England from data derived from primary care records.[16] It is estimated that 4.9% of the population are in stage 3–5 CKD (estimated GFR less than 60 ml/min/1.73m^2), although for methodological reasons this is probably an underestimate.

1.2.1   Is chronic kidney disease a natural consequence of ageing?

For many years glomerular filtration rate has been shown to decline with age. However, is is unclear to what extent these changes are a result of 'normal ageing' or a result of disease processes. The cumulative exposure of the kidney to common causes of chronic kidney disease (atherosclerosis, hypertension, diabetes, heart failure, infection and nephrotoxins) increases with age and it is difficult to separate these from the ageing process.

Only one significant longitudinal study to date has addressed the issue of decreasing GFR with increasing age. In the Baltimore Longitudinal Study of Ageing,[17] 446 community-dwelling participants were followed over a period of up to 24 years. Their data suggests that the decline in GFR with increasing age is largely attributable to hypertension, possibly as a consequence of microvascular disease.[17] In the absence of hypertension or other identifiable causes of renal disease, one-third of older participants were noted to have stable GFR over a period of 20 years. In a small percentage of participants, GFR actually increased with ageing.

Similarly, Fliser et al[18] in a cross-sectional study using inulin clearance found heart failure to be a significant factor in the decline of GFR with increasing age. Additionally, both heart failure and hypertension contributed to reductions in renal plasma flow and increases in the filtration fraction and renal vascular resistance.

In a post-mortem study, Kasiske[19] has demonstrated a relationship between the prevalence of sclerotic glomeruli and atherosclerotic vascular disease. Although twice as many patients with significant atherosclerosis had a history of hypertension as those with milder atherosclerosis, hypertension was not found to be independently predictive of glomerulosclerosis.

Further evidence[20] suggests that cumulative dietary protein intake is an important determinant of the fall in GFR. Studies such as the Antihypertensive and Lipid-Lowering Treatment to Prevent Heart Attack Trial (ALLHAT) have shown that the prevalence of reduced GFR is high in older hypertensive patients. Patients with moderate or severe reduction in GFR in the ALLHAT trial were more likely to have a history of cardiovascular disease and left ventricular hypertrophy compared with those with higher levels of GFR. Even modest reductions in GFR were independently associated with a higher prevalence of cardiovascular disease and left ventricular hypertrophy.[21]

The implications are that disease processes for renal disease in older people are similar to those of younger people and that a decline in renal function is not an inevitable consequence of ageing.

1.2.2 Prevalence of anaemia in patients with chronic kidney disease

The importance of anaemia in CKD has become increasingly apparent since the introduction of erythropoietin treatment into clinical practice in the late 1980s. However, until recently it has not been fully appreciated that anaemia begins to develop early in the course of CKD. NHANES III found lower levels of kidney function to be associated with lower haemoglobin levels and a higher prevalence and severity of anaemia.[22]

Table 1.4 NHANES III data			
eGFR (ml/min/1.73m^2)	Median Hb in men (g/dl)	Median Hb in women (g/dl)	Prevalence of anaemia*
60	14.9	13.5	1%
30	13.8	12.2	9%
15	12.0	10.3	33%

* Hb <12.0 g/dl in men, Hb <11.0 g/dl in women.

The UK information concerning the prevalence of anaemia in patients with CKD comes from two studies. The prevalence of diagnosed CKD, predicated by serum creatinine levels of $\geq$130 µmol/l in women and $\geq$180 µmol/l in men, was 5,554 per million population (pmp), median age was 82 years (range, 18 to 103 years), and median calculated GFR was 28.0 ml/min/1.73m^2 (range, 3.6 to 42.8 ml/min/1.73 m^2).[23] Data for haemoglobin levels were available for 85.6% of patients. Mean haemoglobin concentration was 12.1±1.9 g/dl: 49.6% of men had haemoglobin levels less than 12 g/dl and 51.2% of women had levels less than 11 g/dl. Furthermore, in 27.5% of patients identified, the haemoglobin level was less than 11 g/dl, equivalent to nearly 90,000 of the population based on 2001 Census population figures.

In a larger cross-sectional study abstracting data from 112,215 unselected patients with an age and sex profile representative of the general population, haemoglobin level was weakly correlated with eGFR (r=0.057, p <0.001).[16] The population prevalence of stage 3–5 CKD in this study was estimated to be 4.9%. In those patients with stage 3–5 CKD the prevalence of anaemia, defined as a haemoglobin level less than 12 g/dl in men and post-menopausal women and less than 11 g/dl in pre-menopausal women, was 12.0%, haemoglobin level was less than 11 g/dl in 3.8%, equivalent to over 108,000 of the population based on 2001 Census population figures.

1.2.3   Diabetes, CKD and anaemia

It has been known for some years that anaemia exists in patients with diabetes and CKD, and that this anaemia occurs early in the course of diabetic kidney disease and is associated with inappropriately low erythropoietin concentrations.[24,25] Ishimura et al [25] demonstrated that when those with Type 2 diabetes and CKD are compared with those with non-diabetic CKD, despite similarly advanced CKD and similar serum erythropoietin levels, those with Type 2 diabetes were significantly more anaemic.

Similar findings have also been demonstrated in people with Type 1 diabetes and CKD compared with those without diabetes.[26] More recently, in a series of articles based on cross-sectional surveys of patients with diabetes, Thomas and colleagues demonstrated that at all levels of GFR, anaemia was more prevalent in those with diabetes compared with the general population,[27] that with increasing albuminuria the prevalence of anaemia was higher at each level of renal function,[28] and that levels of erythropoietin were inappropriately low in those with anaemia.[29]

Finally, in a report from the Kidney Early Evaluation Programme (KEEP),[30] the prevalence of anaemia in those with diabetes was significantly higher than in those without diabetes in stage 2 and 3 CKD (7.5% vs 5%, p=0.015 and 22.2% vs 7.9%, p<0.001 respectively). Although the prevalence of anaemia was also higher in those with diabetes in stages 1 and 4 CKD the differences were not significant (8.7% vs 6.9% and 52.4% vs 50% respectively).

1.2.4   Causes of anaemia other than chronic kidney disease

Not all anaemia in patients with CKD will be 'renal anaemia' and causes of anaemia other than CKD should be actively looked for and excluded before a diagnosis of anaemia associated with CKD can be made (Table 1.5)

Table 1.5 Other causes of anaemia in CKD
Chronic blood loss
Iron deficiency
Vitamin B_{12} or folate deficiency
Hypothyroidism
Chronic infection or inflammation
Hyperparathyroidism
Aluminium toxicity
Malignancy
Haemolysis
Bone marrow infiltration
Pure red cell aplasia

Iron deficiency anaemia is the most common cause of anaemia worldwide, either due to negative iron balance through blood loss (commonly gastrointestinal or menstrual), or to inadequate intake which may be nutritional or related to poor gastrointestinal absorption. Studies in elderly patients (aged over 65 years) show that the 'anaemia of chronic disorders' predominates, accounting for 34% to 44% of causes.[31–33]

Iron-deficiency is the cause in 15% to 36% of cases and recent bleeding in 7.3%. Vitamin B_{12} or folate deficiency is the cause in 5.6% to 8.1%, myelodysplastic syndrome and acute leukaemia in 5.6% and chronic leukaemia and lymphoma-related disorders in 5.1%. Other haematological disorders (myelofibrosis, aplastic anaemia, haemolytic anaemia) are the cause in 2.8%, and multiple myeloma in 1.5%.

1.2.5 Pathogenesis of anaemia associated with chronic kidney disease

Although anaemia in patients with CKD may develop in response to a wide variety of causes, erythropoietin deficiency is the primary cause of anaemia associated with CKD. Erythropoietin is predominantly produced by peritubular cells in the kidney and is the hormone responsible for maintaining the proliferation and differentiation of erythroid progenitor cells in the bone marrow. Loss of peritubular cells leads to an inappropriately low level of circulating erythropoietin in the face of anaemia.

Other factors in the genesis of renal anaemia include functional or absolute iron deficiency, blood loss (either occult or overt), the presence of uraemic inhibitors (for example, parathyroid hormone, inflammatory cytokines), reduced half-life of circulating blood cells, and deficiencies of folate or Vitamin B_{12}.

1.3 How to use this guideline

The purpose of this guideline is to support clinical judgement, not to replace it. This means the treating clinician should:

- take into consideration any contraindications in deciding whether or not to administer any treatment recommended by this guideline
- consider the appropriateness of any recommended treatment for a particular patient in terms of the patient's relevant clinical and non-clinical characteristics.

Wherever possible, before administering any treatment the treating clinician should follow good practice in terms of:

- discussing with the patient why the treatment is being offered and what health outcomes are anticipated
- highlighting any possible adverse events or side-effects that have been associated with the treatment
- obtaining explicit consent to administer the treatment.

For those recommendations involving pharmacological treatment, the most recent Summary of Product Characteristics should be followed for the determination of:

- indications
- drug dosage
- method and route of administration
- contraindications
- supervision and monitoring
- product characteristics
- except in those cases where guidance is provided within the recommendation itself.

1.4 Recommendations for children with anaemia of CKD

This guideline gives recommendations for both adults and children. Where the recommendations are different for children, details are given separately, see:

- recommendations R33–35 in section 6.9.6
- recommendation R40 in section 6.12.6.

2 | Methodology

2.1 Aim

The aim of the National Collaborating Centre for Chronic Conditions (NCC-CC) is to provide a user-friendly, clinical, evidence-based guideline for the National Health Service (NHS) that:

- offers best clinical advice for anaemia management in chronic kidney disease (AMCKD)
- is based on best published evidence and expert consensus
- takes into account patient choice and informed decision-making
- defines the major components of NHS care provision for anaemia of CKD
- indicates areas suitable for clinical audit
- details areas of uncertainty or controversy requiring further research
- provides a choice of guideline versions for differing audiences.

2.2 Scope

The guideline was developed in accordance with a scope, which detailed the remit of the guideline originating from the Department of Health and specified those aspects of anaemia of CKD to be included and excluded.

Prior to the commencement of the guideline development, the scope was subjected to stakeholder consultation in accordance with processes established by the National Institute for Health and Clinical Excellence (NICE).[1,34] The full scope is shown in Appendix B.

2.3 Audience

The guideline is intended for use by the following people or organisations:

- all healthcare professionals
- people with anaemia of CKD and their parents and carers
- patient support groups
- commissioning organisations
- service providers.

2.4 Involvement of people with anaemia of CKD

The NCC-CC was keen to ensure the views and preferences of people with anaemia of CKD and their parents and carers informed all stages of the guideline. This was achieved by:

- having a person with anaemia of CKD and a user organisation representative on the Guideline Development Group (GDG)
- consulting the Patient and Public Involvement Programme (PPIP) housed within NICE during the pre-development (scoping) and final validation stages of the guideline.

2.5 Guideline limitations

These include:

- Clinical guidelines usually do not cover issues of **service** delivery, organisation or provision (unless specified in the remit from the Department of Health).
- NICE is primarily concerned with health services and so recommendations are not provided for social services and the voluntary sector. However, the guideline may address important issues in how NHS clinicians interface with these other sectors.
- Generally, the guideline does not cover rare, complex, complicated or unusual conditions.

2.6 Other work relevant to the guideline

The NCC-CC and NICE are developing a clinical guideline on chronic kidney disease (publication is expected in 2008).

NICE has published technology appraisal guidance on erythropoietin for anaemia induced by cancer treatment. This is available from **www.nice.org.uk**

2.7 Background

The development of this evidence-based clinical guideline draws on the methods described by the NICE *Guideline development methods* manual[1] and the methodology pack[35] specifically developed by the NCC-CC for each chronic condition guideline (see **www.rcplondon.ac.uk/college/ncc-cc**). The developers' role and remit is summarised in Table 2.1.

Table 2.1 Role and remit of the developers	
National Collaborating Centre for Chronic Conditions (NCC-CC)	The NCC-CC was set up in 2001 and is housed within the Royal College of Physicians (RCP). The NCC-CC undertakes commissions received from the National Institute for Clinical Excellence (NICE). A multiprofessional partners' board inclusive of patient groups and NHS management governs the NCC-CC.
NCC-CC Technical Team	The technical team met approximately two weeks before each Guideline Development Group (GDG) meeting and comprised the following members: GDG Chair GDG Clinical Advisor Information Scientist Research Fellow Health Economist Project Manager.
Guideline Development Group	The GDG met monthly for 12 months (January to December 2005) and comprised a multidisciplinary team of professionals, service users (a person with anaemia of CKD), carers, and user organisation representatives who were supported by the technical team. The GDG membership details including patient representation and professional groups are detailed in the GDG membership table at the front of this guideline.

continued

Table 2.1 Role and remit of the developers – *continued*	

Guideline Project Executive (PE)	The PE was involved in overseeing all phases of the guideline. It also reviewed the quality of the guideline and compliance with the DH remit and NICE scope.
	
	 The PE comprised:
	     NCC-CC Director
	     NCC-CC Assistant Director
	     NCC-CC Manager
	     NICE Commissioning Manager
	     Technical Team.

Sign-off workshop	At the end of the guideline development process the GDG met to review and agree the guideline recommendations.

Members of the GDG declared any interests in accordance with the NICE technical manual.[1] A register is available from the NCC-CC for inspection upon request: **ncc-cc@rcplondon.ac.uk**

2.8 The process of guideline development

The basic steps in the process of producing a guideline are:

- developing clinical evidence-based questions
- systematically searching for the evidence
- critically appraising the evidence
- incorporating health economic evidence
- distilling and synthesising the evidence and writing recommendations
- grading the evidence statements and recommendations
- agreeing the recommendations
- structuring and writing the guideline
- updating the guideline.

▷ Developing evidence-based questions

The technical team drafted a series of clinical questions that covered the guideline scope. The GDG and Project Executive refined and approved these questions, which are shown in Appendix A.

▷ Searching for the evidence

The information scientist developed a search strategy for each question. Key words for the search were identified by the GDG. In addition, the health economist searched for supplemental papers to inform detailed health economic work (for example modelling). Papers that were published or accepted for publication in peer-reviewed journals were considered as evidence by the GDG. Conference paper abstracts and non-English language papers were excluded from the searches.

Each clinical question dictated the appropriate study design that was prioritised in the search strategy but the strategy was not limited solely to these study types. The research fellow or health economist identified titles and abstracts from the search results that appeared to be relevant to the question. Exclusion lists were generated for each question together with the rationale for the exclusion. The exclusion lists were presented to the GDG. Full papers were obtained where relevant. See Appendix A for literature search details.

▷ Appraising the evidence

The research fellow or health economist, as appropriate, critically appraised the full papers. In general, no formal contact was made with authors, however, there were ad hoc occasions when this was required in order to clarify specific details. Critical appraisal checklists were compiled for each full paper. One research fellow undertook the critical appraisal and data extraction. The evidence was considered carefully by the GDG for accuracy and completeness.

All procedures are fully compliant with:
- NICE methodology as detailed in the '*Guideline development methods – information for National Collaborating Centres and guideline developers*' manual.[1]
- NCC-CC quality assurance document and systematic review chart, available at: **www.rcplondon.ac.uk/college/ncc-cc**

▷ Health economic evidence

Areas for health economic modelling were agreed by the GDG after the formation of the clinical questions. The health economist reviewed the clinical questions to consider the potential application of health economic modelling, and these priorities were agreed with the GDG.

The health economist performed supplemental literature searches to obtain additional data for modelling. Assumptions and designs of the models were explained to and agreed by the GDG members during meetings, and they commented on subsequent revisions.

▷ Distilling and synthesising the evidence and developing recommendations

The evidence from each full paper was distilled into an evidence table and synthesised into evidence statements before being presented to the GDG. This evidence was then reviewed by the GDG and used as a basis on which to formulate recommendations.[2] The criteria for grading evidence and classifying recommendations are shown in Table 2.2.

Evidence tables are available online at **www.rcplondon.ac.uk/college/NCC-CC**

▷ Agreeing the recommendations

The sign-off workshop employed formal consensus techniques[36] to:
- ensure that the recommendations reflected the evidence base
- approve recommendations based on lesser evidence or extrapolations from other situations
- reach consensus recommendations where the evidence was inadequate
- debate areas of disagreement and finalise recommendations.

Table 2.2 Grading the evidence statements and recommendations[2]

Levels of evidence		Classification of recommendations	
Level	**Type of evidence**	**Class**	**Evidence**
1++	High-quality meta-analysis (MA), systematic reviews (SR) of randomised controlled trials (RCTs), or RCTs with a very low risk of bias.	A	Level 1++ and directly applicable to the target population
1+	Well-conducted MA, SR or RCTs, or RCTs with a low risk of bias.		*or* Level 1+ and directly applicable to the target population **AND** consistency of results. Evidence from NICE technology appraisal.
1−	MA, SR of RCTs, or RCTs with a high risk of bias.		Not used as a basis for making a recommendation.
2++	High-quality SR of case-control or cohort studies. High-quality case-control or cohort studies with a very low risk of confounding, bias or chance and a high probability that the relationship is causal.	B	Level 2++, directly applicable to the target population and demonstrating overall consistency of results. *or* Extrapolated evidence from 1++ or 1+.
2+	Well-conducted case-control or cohort studies with a low risk of confounding, bias or chance and a moderate probability that the relationship is causal.		
2−	Case-control or cohort studies with a high risk of confounding, bias or chance and a significant risk that the relationship is not causal		Not used as a basis for making a recommendation.
3	Non-analytic studies (for example case reports, case series).	C	Level 2+, directly applicable to the target population and demonstrating overall consistency of results *or* Extrapolated evidence from 2++.
4	Expert opinion, formal consensus.	D	Level 3 or 4 *or* Extrapolated from 2+ *or* Formal consensus.
		GPP	A good practice point (GPP) is a recommendation based on the experience of the GDG.

Diagnostic study level of evidence and classification of recommendation was also included.[1]

The sign-off workshop also reached agreement on the following:
- five to ten key priorities for implementation
- five key research recommendations
- algorithms.

In prioritising key recommendations for implementation, the sign-off workshop also took into account the following criteria:

- high clinical impact
- high impact on reducing variation
- more efficient use of NHS resources
- allowing the patient to reach critical points in the care pathway more quickly.

The audit criteria provide suggestions of areas for audit in line with the key recommendations for implementation.[1]

▷ Structuring and writing the guideline

The guideline is divided into sections for ease of reading. For each section the layout is similar and contains:

- *Clinical introduction* sets a succinct background and describes the current clinical context.
- *Methodological introduction* describes any issues or limitations that were apparent when reading the evidence base.
- *Evidence statements* provide a synthesis of the evidence base and usually describe what the evidence showed in relation to the outcomes of interest.
- *Health economics* presents, where appropriate, an overview of the cost-effectiveness evidence base.
- *From evidence to recommendations* sets out the GDG decision-making rationale providing a clear and explicit audit trail from the evidence to the evolution of the recommendations.
- *Recommendations* provide stand alone, action-orientated recommendations.
- *Evidence tables* are not published as part of the full guideline but are available online at **www.rcplondon.ac.uk/college/NCC-CC** These describe comprehensive details of the primary evidence that was considered during the writing of each section.

▷ Writing the guideline

The first draft version of the guideline was drawn up by the technical team in accord with the decision of the GDG. The guideline was then submitted for two formal rounds of public and stakeholder consultation prior to publication.[1] The registered stakeholders for this guideline are detailed on the NICE website, see **www.nice.org.uk**. Editorial responsibility for the full guideline rests with the GDG.

The following versions of the guideline are available:

Table 2.3 Versions of this guideline	
Full version	Details the recommendations. The supporting evidence base and the expert considerations of the GDG. Available at **www.rcplondon.ac.uk/pubs/books/AMCKD/**
NICE version	Documents the recommendations without any supporting evidence. Available at **www.nice.org.uk/page.aspx?o=guidelines.completed**
Quick reference guide	An abridged version. Available at **www.nice.org.uk/page.aspx?o=guidelines.completed**
Information for the public	A lay version of the guideline recommendations. Available at **www.nice.org.uk/page.aspx?o=guidelines.completed**

▷ Updating the guideline

Literature searches were repeated for all of the evidence-based questions at the end of the GDG development process, allowing any relevant papers published by 28 September 2005 to be considered. Future guideline updates will consider evidence published after this cut-off date.

Two years after publication of the guideline, NICE will commission a National Collaborating Centre to determine whether the evidence base has progressed significantly to alter the guideline recommendations and warrant an early update. If not, the guideline will be updated approximately 4 years after publication.[1]

2.9 Disclaimer

Healthcare providers need to use clinical judgement, knowledge and expertise when deciding whether it is appropriate to apply guidelines. The recommendations cited here are a guide and may not be appropriate for use in all situations. The decision to adopt any of the recommendations cited here must be made by the practitioner in light of individual patient circumstances, the wishes of the patient, clinical expertise and resources.

The NCC-CC disclaims any responsibility for damages arising out of the use or non-use of these guidelines and the literature used in support of these guidelines.

2.10 Funding

The National Collaborating Centre for Chronic Conditions was commissioned by the National Institute for Health and Clinical Excellence to undertake the work on this guideline.

3 | Key messages of the guideline

3.1 Key priorities for implementation

Management of anaemia should be considered in people with anaemia of chronic kidney disease (CKD) when the haemoglobin level is less than or equal to 11g/dl (or 10 g/dl if under 2 years of age).

Treatment with erythropoiesis stimulating agents (ESAs) should be offered to patients with anaemia of CKD who are likely to benefit in terms of quality of life and physical function.

ESA therapy should be clinically effective, consistent and safe in people with anaemia of CKD. To achieve this, the prescriber and patient should agree a plan which is patient-centred and includes:

- continuity of drug supply
- flexibility of where the drug is delivered and administered
- the lifestyle and preferences of the patient
- cost of drug supply
- desire for self-care where appropriate
- regular review of the plan in light of changing needs.

In people with anaemia of CKD, treatment should maintain stable haemoglobin (Hb) levels between 10.5 and 12.5 g/dl for adults and children aged over 2 years, and between 10 and 12 g/dl in children aged under 2 years, reflecting the lower normal range in that age group. This should be achieved by:

- considering adjustments to treatment, typically when Hb rises above 12.0 or falls below 11.0 g/dl
- taking patient preferences, symptoms and comorbidity into account and revising the aspirational range and action thresholds accordingly.

Age alone should not be a determinant for treatment of anaemia of CKD.

People receiving ESA maintenance therapy should be given iron supplements to keep their:
- serum ferritin between 200 and 500 µg/l in both haemodialysis patients and non-haemodialysis patients, **and either**
    - the transferrin saturation level above 20% (unless ferritin >800 ug/l) **or**
    - percentage hypochromic red cells (%HRC) less than 6% (unless ferritin >800ug/l).

In practice it is likely this will require intravenous iron.

3.2 Algorithms

An algorithm is any set of detailed instructions which results in a predictable end-state from a known beginning, ideally presented in an easy-to-follow decision tree format. Algorithms are only as good as the instructions given, however, and the result will be incorrect if the algorithm is not properly defined. The algorithms presented in this section are suggested management algorithms based on the known literature but importantly they have not been tested and should be used as guides to aid development of local practice.

3.2.1 Algorithm for diagnosis of anaemia of CKD in adults

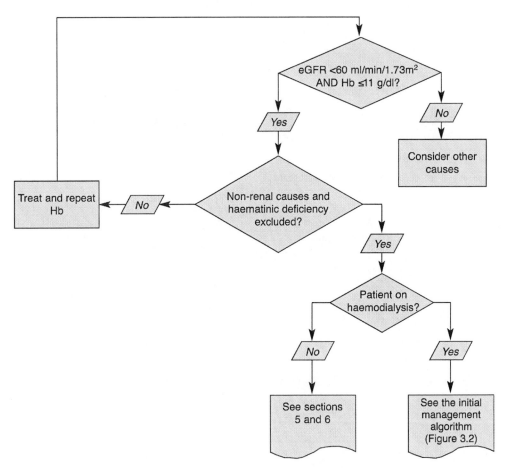

Figure 3.1 Diagnosis of anaemia of CKD in adults

Table 3.1 Test for functional iron deficiency with ferritin and TSAT or ferritin and %HRC				
	Ferritin	**TSAT %**	**MCV**	**HRC %**
Functional iron deficiency	>100 µg/l	<20	Normal range	>6
Absolute iron deficiency	<100 µg/l	<20	Low	>6
TSAT = transferrin saturation; MCV = mean corpuscular volume; HRC = hypochromic red cells.				

3.2.2 Initial management algorithm for adult patients (assumes Hb <11g/dl)

This algorithm is an example strategy for adult haemodialysis patients. Treatment should be tailored to individual patients according to the guideline recommendations.

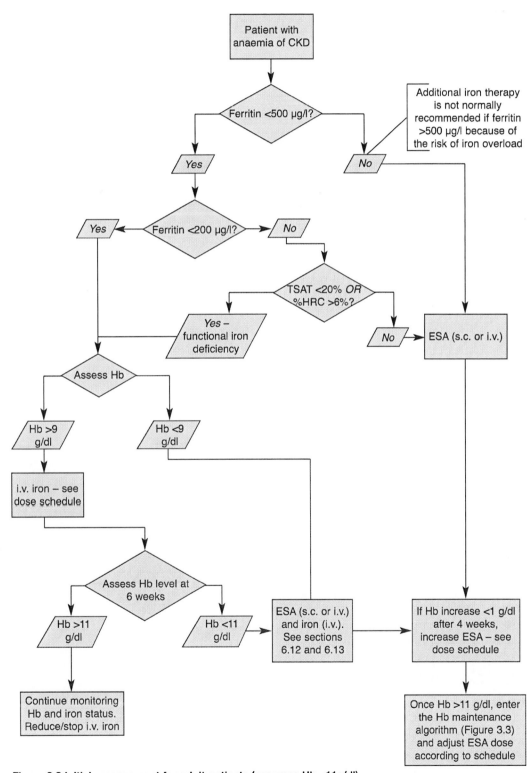

Figure 3.2 Initial management for adult patients (assumes Hb <11g/dl)

▷ Iron dosage schedule

This is an example strategy for adult haemodialysis patients weighing over 50 kg. Treatment should be tailored to individual patients according to the guideline recommendations.

Table 3.2 Iron dosage schedule

Haemodialysis patients		Non-haemodialysis patients
Induction/loading dose	**Maintenance dose**	Iron sucrose 200 mg/fortnight x 3 doses or low molecular weight iron dextran 1g
Either iron sucrose 200 mg/week for 5 weeks or low molecular weight iron dextran 1g	Iron sucrose 50 mg/week or 100 mg/fortnight	

Throughout ESA induction:

In people with anaemia of chronic kidney disease, haemoglobin should be monitored:

● every 2–4 weeks in the induction phase of ESA therapy

● every 1–3 months in the maintenance phase of ESA therapy

● more actively after an ESA dose adjustment

● in a clinical setting chosen in discussion with the patient, taking into consideration their convenience and local healthcare systems.

Be aware of side effects and comorbidities

3.2.3 Haemoglobin maintenance algorithm (assumes patient is receiving ESA and maintenance i.v. iron)

This is an example strategy for adult patients. Treatment should be tailored to individual patients according to the guideline recommendations.

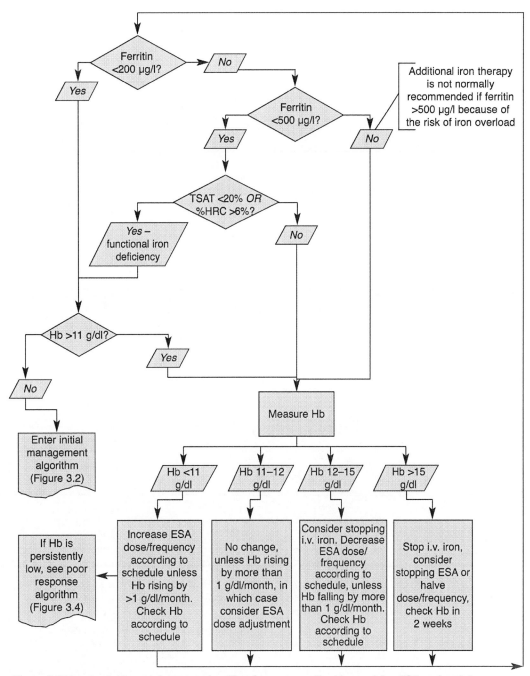

Figure 3.3 Haemoglobin maintenance algorithm (assumes patient is receiving ESA and maintenance i.v. iron)

▷ ESA adjustment schedule for adult patients – make adjustments based on absolute Hb level and/or rate of change of Hb >1g/dl/month

Table 3.3 Erythropoietins

Current dose (units/week)	Increased dose (if single dose consider increasing dose frequency)	Decreased dose (consider reducing dose frequency, minimum weekly)
1,000	2,000	Suspend
2,000	3,000	1,000
3,000	4,000	2,000
4,000	6,000	3,000
6,000	9,000	4,000
9,000	12,000	6,000
12,000	Seek advice	9,000
>12,000	Seek advice	Seek advice

Table 3.4 Darbepoetin

Current dose (µg/week)	Increased dose (consider increasing dose frequency)	Decreased dose (consider reducing dose frequency, minimum monthly)
10	15	Suspend
15	20	10
20	30	15
30	40	20
40	50	30
50	60	40
60	80	50
80	Seek advice	60
>80	Seek advice	Seek advice

▷ Frequency of haemoglobin monitoring in adults

Table 3.5 Haemodialysis patients

Haemoglobin level and rate of change	Monitoring frequency
<11 g/dl, rate of change ≤1 g/dl/month	4 weeks
<11 g/dl, rate of change >1 g/dl/month	2 weeks
11–12 g/dl, rate of change ≤1 g/dl/month	4 weeks
11–12 g/dl, rate of change >1 g/dl/month	2 weeks
>12–15 g/dl, rate of change ≤1 g/dl/month	4 weeks
>12–15 g/dl, rate of change >1 g/dl/month	2 weeks
>15 g/dl	2 weeks

Table 3.6 Peritoneal dialysis and predialysis (including transplant) patients

<11 g/dl, rate of change ≤1 g/dl/month	4 weeks
<11 g/dl, rate of change >1 g/dl/month	2 weeks
11–12 g/dl, rate of change ≤1 g/dl/month	4–12 weeks
11–12 g/dl, rate of change >1 g/dl/month	2 weeks
>12–15 g/dl, rate of change ≤1 g/dl/month	4–12 weeks
>12–15 g/dl, rate of change >1 g/dl/month	2 weeks
>15 g/dl	2 weeks

3.2.4   Algorithm for adult patients with poor response to ESAs

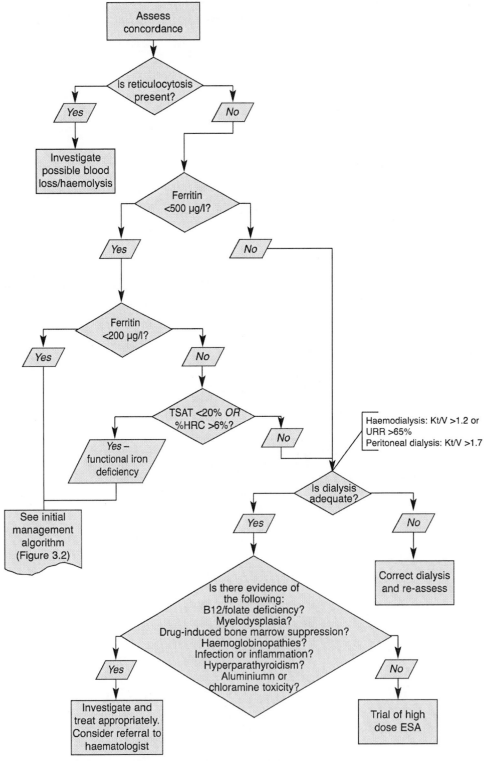

Figure 3.4 Algorithm for adult patients with poor response to ESAs

3.3 Audit criteria

Table 3.7 Audit criteria		
Key priority for implementation	**Criterion**	**Exception**
Management of anaemia should be considered in people with anaemia of chronic kidney disease (CKD) when the haemoglobin level is less than or equal to 11 g/dl (or 10 g/dl if under 2 years of age).	1. % of patients with CKD with recorded Hb ≤11 g/dl (or 10 g/dl if under 2 years of age) who were started on iron/ESAs at the time, or at the following appointment.	Documented refusal, contraindications.
Treatment with ESAs should be offered to patients with anaemia of CKD who are likely to benefit in terms of quality of life and physical function.	2. % of patients with ACKD with recorded Hb ≤11 g/dl not on anaemia treatment, with a breakdown of the reasons for it not being offered.	
ESA therapy should be clinically effective, consistent and safe in people with anaemia of CKD. To achieve this, the prescriber and patient should agree a plan which is patient-centred and includes: • provision of a secure drug supply • flexibility of where the drug is delivered and administered • lifestyle and preferences • cost of drug supply • desire for self-care where appropriate • regular review of the plan in light of changing needs.	3. % of patients with ACKD receiving anaemia treatment who are receiving ESAs, with a plan recorded as specified.	
In people with anaemia of chronic kidney disease, treatment should maintain stable haemoglobin (Hb) levels between 10.5 and 12.5 g/dl for adults and children aged over 2 years, and between 10 and 12 g/dl in children aged under 2 years, reflecting the lower normal range in that age group. This should be achieved by: • Considering adjustments to treatment, typically when Hb rises above 12.0 or falls below 11.0 g/dl. • Taking patient preferences, symptoms and comorbidity into account and revising the aspirational range and action thresholds accordingly.	4. % of patients with diagnosed ACKD who have received treatment for 3 months or longer and, at the time of a cross-sectional audit, have Hb levels between 10.5 and 12.5 g/dl for adults and children aged over 2 years, or between 10 and 12 g/dl in children aged under 2 years.	Patients who have underlying causes for poor response (see section 1.2.4), patients who are in the induction phase of their treatment.
		continued

Table 3.7 Audit criteria – *continued*

Key priority for implementation	Criterion	Exception
Patients receiving ESA maintenance therapy should be given iron supplements to keep their: • serum ferritin between 200 and 500 µg/l in both haemodialysis patients and non-haemodialysis patients, **and either** • the transferrin saturation level above 20% (unless ferritin > 800 ug/l) **or** • percentage hypochromic red cells (%HRC) less than 6% (unless ferritin > 800ug/l). In practice it is likely this will require i.v. iron.	5. % of patients with diagnosed ACKD and on maintenance therapy with ESAs who, at the time of a cross-sectional audit, have: • serum ferritin between 200 and 500 µg/l in both haemodialysis patients and non-haemodialysis patients **and either** • The transferrin saturation level above 20% (unless ferritin >800 ug/l) **or** • percentage hypochromic red cells (%HRC) less than 6% (unless ferritin >800ug/l).	

THE GUIDELINE

4 | Diagnostic evaluation and assessment of anaemia

4.1 Diagnostic role of Hb levels

4.1.1 Clinical introduction

Possible adverse effects of anaemia in patients with CKD include reduced oxygen utilisation, increased cardiac output and left ventricular hypertrophy (cardiac dilatation ± increased wall thickness). The relationships between these are set out in Figure 4.1.

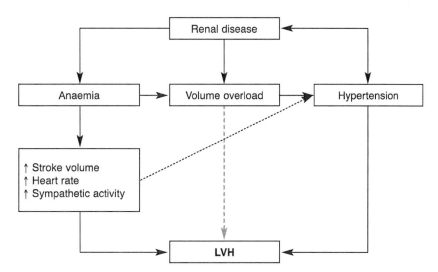

Figure 4.1 Left ventricular hypertrophy (LVH) in CKD patients (Mann JF, *Nephrol Dial Transplant* 1999;14(Suppl 2):29–36)

It is also suggested that anaemia is associated with increased progression of CKD, reduced cognition and concentration, reduced libido and reduced immune responsiveness. How much these adverse effects translate into adverse outcomes such as impaired quality of life, increased hospitalisation, increased cardiovascular events and increased cardiovascular and all-cause mortality has been the subject of debate for several years.

Large observational studies show an inverse association between haemoglobin levels and adverse outcomes but randomised controlled trial (RCT) evidence of an improvement in these outcomes with correction of anaemia is lacking. Part of the problem is that the available studies do not compare 'no treatment of anaemia' with treatment, but rather partial correction of anaemia to better correction.

Is it likely that adverse outcomes associated with anaemia are influenced by age, gender or ethnicity? The implications of this question are that we might adopt a differing strategy when correcting anaemia if there is evidence to dictate such an approach.

4.1.2 Methodological introduction

A literature search identified longitudinal,[37–40] before and after[41–44] and cohort[45–48] studies, conducted predominantly in haemodialysis patients.

Four studies[49–52] had methodological limitations and were excluded from evidence statements.

Notable aspects of the evidence base were:

- No studies were found which specifically addressed the issues of gender and ethnicity and only one study was identified which stratified the study population according to age.[44]
- Only two studies included populations over 80 years old.[38,47]
- Not all studies reported gender and ethnicity of the participants. Some studies included predominantly male[42,43] or predominantly white participants[46,47] or predominantly male and white participants.[48,50] One study included a population that was 67% African American.[38]
- The number of study participants varied greatly, ranging between 7 and over 60,000.

A comprehensive literature search did not identify any studies that were suitable to address the economic aspects, therefore no health economic evidence statements are given.

4.1.3 Evidence statements

These evidence statements are grouped by outcome measure per sub-population of anaemia patients.

▷ Left ventricular hypertrophy

Predialysis patients

In a 1-year study (n=318),[48] a mean decrease in Hb of 0.5 g/dl from baseline of 12.8 ± 1.9 g/dl was found to be one of three factors (including systolic blood pressure and left ventricular (LV) mass index) that was associated with left ventricular hypertrophy (LVH) (OR 1.32, 95% CI 1.1 to 1.59, p=0.004). (**Level 2+**)

A decrease in LV mass index (p<0.01) was observed after raising haematocrit (Hct) from 23.6 ± 0.5% (Hb ~ 7.8 g/dl) to 39.1 ± 0.8% (Hb ~ 13 g/dl) with epoetin over a time period of 12 months in a small sample (n=9).[41] Similarly, in another study (n=11)[37] treatment with epoetin increased Hct levels from 26.3 ± 0.6% (Hb ~ 8.7 g/dl) to 34.4 ± 1.1% (Hb ~ 11.4 g/dl) at 3 months and 34.7 ± 1.3% (Hb ~ 11.5 g/dl) at 6 months. A reduction in LV mass index at month 6 (p<0.05), cardiac output (p<0.05), cardiac index (p<0.05), and an increase in total peripheral resistance (p<0.05) at months 3 and 6 of the study were observed. (**Level 3**)

In two studies,[37,41] increased Hct levels with epoetin from 26.3 ± 0.6% (Hb ~ 8.7 g/dl) to 34.7 ± 1.3% (Hb ~ 11.5 g/dl) at 6 months[37] and from 23.6 ± 0.5% (Hb ~ 7.8 g/dl) to 39.1 ± 0.8% (Hb ~ 13 g/dl) at 12 months[41] found no changes in LV end-diastolic/systolic diameters, interventricular septum thickness, LV posterior wall thickness over 6 months[37] or over 12 months.[41] (**Level 3**)

Haemodialysis patients

In a 12 month study[42] where Hb was increased from a baseline level of 6.3 ± 0.8 g/dl to 11.4 ± 1.5 g/dl by epoetin administration, a reduction in LV mass (p <0.001), LV end-diastolic volume (p=0.005) and LV end diastole (p=0.003) was found in patients with baseline LV mass above 210 g. In the same study,[42] no significant changes were observed in echocardiography measurements of LV posterior wall, interventricular septum or mean wall thickness. (**Level 3**)

In a small study (n=7),[43] an increase in Hb from 9.8 ± 1.3 g/dl to 14.2 ± 0.6 g/dl using epoetin over a period of approximately 6 months found a significant reduction in cardiac output (p<0.01) and stroke volume (p<0.01), which was accompanied with a significant increase in total peripheral resistance (p<0.05). However, there was no change in mean arterial pressure. (**Level 3**)

▷ Hospitalisation

Haemodialysis patients

A cohort (n=66,761), with data stratified into increasing Hct levels and compared with an Hct level of 33 to 35% over a 1-year follow-up period[46] found the following:

Table 4.1 Summary data from study[46] (Level 2+)					
Hct (%)	**<30**	**30 to 32**	**33 to 35 (Ref)**	**36 to 38**	**≥39**
Hb (g/dl)	**<10**	**10-10.7**	**11 to 11.7 (Ref)**	**12 to 12.7**	**≥13**
RR of all-cause hospitalisation	1.42	1.21	1	0.78	0.84
RR of hospitalisation from cardiac causes	1.3	1.17	1	0.75	NS
RR of hospitalisation from infections	1.76	1.3	1	0.82	0.62

RR = relative risk; NS = not significant.

In a 2.5-year follow-up study,[47] participants (n=50,579) were stratified into increasing Hct levels and compared with patients with the arbitrary reference of Hct 34 to 36% (n=22,192), see Tables 4.2 to 4.5.

Table 4.2 Adjusted relative risk of first hospitalisation due to any cardiac disease[47] (Level 2+)					
Hct (%)	**≤30**	**31 to 33**	**34 to 36 (Ref)**	**37 to 39**	**≥40**
Hb (g/dl)	**≤10**	**10.3 to 11**	**11.3 to 12 (Ref)**	**12.3 to 13**	**≥13.3**
RR	1.18	1.07	1.00	0.92	0.79
95% CI	Not reported	Not reported	N/A	0.88 to 0.97	0.72 to 0.87

RR = relative risk.

Table 4.3 Adjusted relative risk of first hospitalisation due to specific cardiac diseases[47] (Level 2+)

Hct (%)	34 to 36 (Ref)	37 to 39	≥40
Hb (g/dl)	11.3 to 12 (Ref)	12.3 to 13	≥13.3
RR due to congestive heart failure, fluid overload or cardiomyopathy	1.00	0.85 (95% CI 0.77 to 0.95)	0.80 (95% CI 0.65 to 0.97)
RR due to ischemic heart disease, cerebrovascular disease or circulatory system disease	1.00	NS	0.81 (95% CI 0.70 to 0.93)
RR due to other cardiac diseases	1.00	NS	0.76 (95% CI 0.62 to 0.92)

RR = relative risk; NS = not significant.

Table 4.4 Adjusted relative risk of first hospitalisation for patients with cardiac comorbid conditions (n=45,166)[47] (Level 2+)

Hct (%)	34 to 36	37 to 39	≥40
Hb (g/dl)	11.3 to 12	12.3 to 13	≥13.3
Relative risk	1.00	0.93	0.79
95% CI	N/A	0.89 to 0.98	0.71 to 0.87

Table 4.5 Adjusted relative risk of hospitalisation for patients with Hct 37 to 39% without pre-existing cardiac disease (3-year follow-up)[47] (Level 2+)

	RR	p value
All-cause hospitalisation	0.78	<0.0001
Any cardiac hospitalisation	0.74	0.0005

▷ Mortality

Haemodialysis patients

Data from a cohort (n=66,761) were stratified into increasing Hct levels and compared with an arbitrary Hct level of 33 to 35% over a 1-year follow-up period:[46]

Table 4.6 Adjusted relative risks (Level 2+)

Hct (%)	<30	30 to 32	33 to 35 (Ref)	36 to 38	≥39
Hb (g/dl)	<10	10-10.7	11 to 11.7 (Ref)	12 to 12.7	≥13
RR of all-cause mortality	1.74	1.25	1	NS	NS
RR of mortality from cardiac causes	1.57	1.25	1	NS	NS
RR of mortality from infections	1.92	1.26	1	NS	NS

NS = not significant.

In a 3-year follow-up study[47] participants (n=50,579) were stratified into Hct levels and compared with patients with the arbitrary reference of Hct 34 to 36% (n=22,192):

Table 4.7 Adjusted relative risk of mortality due to cardiac diseases[47]

Hct (%)	34 to 36 (Ref)	37 to 39	≥40
Hb (g/dl)	11.3 to 12 (Ref)	12.3 to 13	≥13.3
Relative risk	1.00	0.92	0.83
95% CI	N/A	0.87 to 0.98	0.74 to 0.93

Table 4.8 Adjusted relative risk of all-cause mortality[47]

Hct (%)	34 to 36 (Ref)	37 to 39	≥40
Hb (g/dl)	11.3 to 12 (Ref)	12.3 to 13	≥13.3
Relative risk	1.00	0.92	0.86
95% CI	N/A	0.88 to 0.96	0.80 to 0.93

Table 4.9 Adjusted relative risk of mortality for patients with Hct 37 to 39% without pre-existing cardiac disease[47]

	RR	p value
All-cause death	0.69	0.0002
Any cardiac death	0.69	0.0137

In one study (n=309),[38] no association was found between any Hct quartile (<33.4%, ≥33.4 to 35.73%, ≥35.74% to 38.55%, and >38.55%) and survival over 18 months. (**Level 3**)

In a 4-year study,[39] renal units with more than 87% of patients achieving target Hct ≥33% (Hb ≥11 g/dl) had a lower mortality rate than those with less than 64% of patients achieving target Hct (p<0.0001). A 10% point increase in the fraction of patients with Hct of more than or equal to 33% (Hb ≥11 g/dl) was found to be associated with a 1.5% decrease in mortality (p=0.003). (**Level 3**)

A retrospective cohort study with 1-year follow-up (n=75,283)[45] found an increase in the age group associated with higher all-cause and cause-specific mortality. Female patients had better outcomes. When compared with white patients, black patients and other ethnic minority patients had lower all-cause and cause-specific mortality. In the same study,[45] mortality data were compared with Hct 30 to <33% (Hb 10 to <11 g/dl),[45] see Table 4.10.

Table 4.10 Adjusted relative risks[47] (Level 2+)					
Hct (%)	**<27** **(n=9,130)**	**27 to <30** **(n=22,217)**	**30 to <33 (REF)** **(n=33,122)**	**33 to <36** **(n=10,129)**	**1992 and 1993 data** **33 to <36 (n=61,797)**
Hb	**<9 g/dl** **(n=9,130)**	**9 to <10 g/dl** **(n=22,217)**	**10 to <11 g/dl** **(REF) (n=33,122)**	**11 to <12 g/dl** **(n=10,129)**	**1992 & 1993 data** **11 to <12 g/dl** **(n=61,797)**
RR of all-cause death	1.33 95% CI 1.26–1.40	1.13 95% CI 1.08–1.17	1.00	NS	0.96 95% CI 0.92–0.99
RR of cardiac death	1.25 95% CI 1.15–1.35	1.11 95% CI 1.05–1.17	1.00	NS	Not reported
RR of infectious death	1.53 95% CI 1.33–2.75	1.13 95% CI 1.02–1.26	1.00	NS	Not reported

NS = not significant.

▷ MI, stroke and all-cause mortality

Predialysis patients

In one study (n=2,333),[40] the hazard ratio for the composite outcome (MI, stroke and all-cause mortality) was significantly increased in individuals with anaemia (defined as Hb <12 g/dl or Hct <36% in women and Hb <13 g/dl or Hct <39% in men) when compared with those without anaemia (hazard ratio 1.51; 95% CI 1.27 to 1.81). (**Level 3**)

▷ Quality of life

Haemodialysis patients

When evaluated in epoetin-treated patients (n=57)[44] whose Hct increased from 21 ± 0.3% (Hb ~ 7 g/dl) at baseline to 28 ± 0.4% (Hb ~ 9.3 g/dl) at month 3 and 29 ± 0.4% (Hb ~ 9.7 g/dl) at month 6, quality of life was shown to improve by means of the Karnofsky scale (p=0.0001) and the global (p=0.0001), physical (p=0.0001) and psychosocial (p=0.0001) dimensions of the Sickness Impact Profile (SIP) questionnaire. This was further reinforced by linear regression between improvement of the SIP global score and final achieved Hct (29 ± 0.4%) (b coefficient 0.57, p<0.05, R^2 0.57). (**Level 2+**)

▷ Effect of age on quality of life

Haemodialysis patients

In a subgroup analysis of epoetin-treated patients divided into age groups of more than or equal to 60 years (n=23) and less than 60 years (n=34), Hct levels were higher in the younger age group (p<0.05).[44] No differences were observed in improvements of quality of life scores using the Karnofsky scale or SIP score when these age groups were compared.[44] The same was true when patients were stratified into age groups of more than 60 years (n=34) and more than or equal to 65 years (n=15).[44] (**Level 2+**)

4.1.4 From evidence to recommendations

Data about the outcome of LVH were presented to the GDG.[48] Two studies which demonstrated an association between decreasing left ventricular mass and increasing haematocrit levels[37,41] were based on small sample sizes (n=9 and n=11) and the GDG weighed these studies accordingly in their deliberations.

Two studies were appraised that examined the rate of progression of renal failure but these were excluded as underpowered by the GDG[37,41] and hence, no evidence statements were presented for this outcome.

The GDG noted that the greater hospitalisation rate seen in a study based on registry data[46] could be a reflection of a sicker population and this may be another reason for the lower Hb level. It was also noted that the lowest haematocrit group required double the amount of EPO to reach this level, and as such, these participants may have a reduced health status.

The study by Moreno et al [49] was excluded by the GDG because of a highly selected population (excluding both elderly and ill patients) and a lack of intention to treat analysis. The group agreed to increase the grade of one other study[47] from 3 to 2+ as the study participants had been subdivided according to Hct levels and a multivariate analysis of risk had been performed.

The GDG agreed that the evidence supported an association between decreased haematocrit and increased risk of hospitalisation.

The group felt that the evidence presented on mortality from one study[46] suggested that there was an increase in mortality between Hct <30 to <33% (Hb levels ~ 1 –11g/dl) when compared with Hct 33 to 36% (Hb ~ 11–12g/dl). It was noted that this range spans the standard levels quoted in many guidelines. The data presented by two studies[39,45] suggest that a Hb of <11g/dl was the threshold below which there was an increased risk of mortality. However, the GDG noted that these studies may not have accounted for confounding factors such as intercurrent illness. The issue was also raised that there might be a reverse causality and that patients requiring high amounts of epoetin may be sicker and hence more likely to require hospitalisation.

One study[38] concluded that the haematocrit level was not a predictor of survival and that other markers of morbidity were more important. The data also suggested that confounding factors may be present that were not taken into account, eg infection. This possibility was reflected in the study as the haematocrit levels were corrected for albumin. This study also suggested that men and women require different doses of ESA: women appear to need more ESA than men.

Only one study was appraised that evaluated haemodynamic parameters but this was excluded for this outcome by the GDG as it was felt to be underpowered (n=7).[43]

Concerning quality of life in haemodialysis patients(n=57),[44] a subgroup analysis of those over and under 60 years of age found a significant increase in quality of life scores associated with higher Hb levels in both age groups.

RECOMMENDATION

R1   Management of anaemia should be considered in people with anaemia of chronic kidney disease (CKD) when their haemoglobin level is less than or equal to 11 g/dl **(C)** (or 10 g/dl if younger than 2 years of age).   **(D)**

See 3.2.1 for the associated algorithm.

4.2   Diagnostic role of glomerular filtration rate

4.2.1   Clinical introduction

Data from population studies such as NHANES III in the USA and the NEOERICA study in the UK suggest an increasing prevalence of anaemia with decreasing GFR level. A similar relationship between glomerular filtration rate (GFR) and anaemia has also been demonstrated in population cohorts of people with diabetes.[27] Although anaemia is common in people with diabetes it is also commonly unrecognised and undetected.[53] The prevalence of anaemia in people with diabetes is increased at all levels of renal function in those with increased proteinuria/albuminuria,[54] and it has been suggested that in people with diabetes, anaemia associated with CKD may occur earlier in the evolution of CKD when compared with people without diabetes. In investigating the evidence base, this section seeks to describe the relationship between GFR and haemoglobin levels and provide guidance for clinicians about the threshold level of GFR below which they should suspect that anaemia is associated with CKD.

4.2.2   Methodological introduction

A literature search identified five studies investigating the association between GFR or creatinine clearance (CCr) with Hb/Hct levels in non-diabetic patients[55–59] and four studies in diabetic patients.[16,27,28,30]

Notable aspects of the evidence base were:

- Two studies were not limited to patients with CKD.[55,56]
- Two studies were conducted in selected patient populations[57,58] and one study[59] was conducted in children.
- Patient populations in some studies were not stratified to diabetic and non-diabetic patients and where reported, the percentage of diabetics varied from 5%[55] to 28%[58] and to 64.4%.[57] All patients with CKD were in the untreated predialysis stage, except for one study where some patients received oral iron (26%) and epoetin (12.8%) to treat their anaemia.[59]
- One study was conducted in people with Type 2 diabetes,[28] and one in people with Type 1 and people with Type 2 diabetes.[27]

A comprehensive literature search did not identify any studies that were suitable to address the economic aspects, therefore no health economic evidence statements are given.

4.2.3 Evidence statements

▷ Hb/Hct levels associated with different GFR or CCr levels in non-diabetic patients

Table 4.11 GFR vs Hb[55] (Level 3)

Median Hb level in women (g/dl)	Median Hb level in men (g/dl)	eGFR (ml/min/1.73 m^2)
13.5	14.9	60
12.2	13.8	30
10.3	12.0	15

Table 4.12 GFR vs Hb using >80 ml/min/1.73 m^2 as the reference value[56] (Level 2+)

GFR (ml/min/1.73 m^2) >80=ref	Women (n=8,495)		Men (n=3,560)	
	Difference in Hb (g/dl)	p value	Difference in Hb (g/dl)	p value
>70 to ≤80	0.1 95% CI 0.1–0.2	<0.0001	NS	0.44
>60 to ≤70	0.1 95% CI 0.1–0.2	0.0009	NS	0.40
>50 to ≤60	0.1 95% CI 0.0–0.2	0.006	-0.2 95% CI -0.3–0.0	0.07
>40 to ≤50	-0.2 95% CI -0.4, -0.1	0.0004	-0.8 95% CI -1.1, -0.5	<0.0001
>30 to ≤40	-0.6 95% CI -0.8, -0.3	<0.0001	-1.4 95% CI -1.8, -1.0	<0.0001
>20 to ≤30	-1.4 95% CI -1.8, -1.1	<0.0001	-1.9 95% CI -2.3, -1.4	<0.0001
≤20	-1.9 95% CI -2.3, -1.6	<0.0001	-3.4 95% CI -3.9, -2.9	<0.0001

Table 4.13 GFR vs Hb[57] (Level 3)

GFR (ml/min/1.73m²)	n	% of n with Hb ≤10 g/dl	% of n with Hb >10 to ≤12 g/dl	% of n with Hb ≤12 g/dl
≥60	116	5.2	21.6	26.7
≥30 to <60	2,832	5.6	35.9	41.6
≥15 to <30	1,968	11.0	42.6	53.6
<15	298	27.2	48.3	75.5

Table 4.14 GFR vs Hct[58] (Level 2+)

Hct (%)	Estimated Hb (g/dl)	GFR (ml/min/1.73 m²)
<28	<9	16.5 ± 6.8
28.0–29.9	9–<10	17.9 ± 8.8
30.0–32.9	10–<11	20.1 ± 7.6
33.0–35.9	11–<12	22.0 ± 8.9
≥36	≥12	27.4 ± 7.9

Table 4.15 GFR vs Hct in children (<21 years old)[59]

	% of patients with Hct		
	≤30 %	31–32.9 %	>33 %
	% of patients with estimated Hb (g/dl)		
	≤10	>10–<11	>11
All patients	30.9 %	13.0 %	56.1 %
GFR (ml/min/1.73 m²)			
<10	62.9 %	11.3 %	25.8 %
10–25	48.1 %	16.8 %	35.1 %
25–50	25.7 %	13.3 %	61.0 %
50–75	13.1 %	8.1 %	78.7 %

2.4% of the study participants were treated with RBC transfusions after study entry. In addition, 26% of study participants received oral iron and 12.8% received epoetin during the course of the study. (**Level 2+**)

▷ Hb levels associated with different GFR levels in diabetic patients

In a retrospective cross-sectional study (n=28,862),[16] diabetes was recorded in 15.4% of patients with GFR of more than 60 (stage 3–5 CKD). Of these, 15.3% were anaemic when defined as Hb <12 g/dl for women and <13 g/dl for men) and 3.8% were anaemic when defined as Hb <11 g/dl. (**Level 3**)

In a retrospective cross-sectional study in people with Type 1 and 2 diabetes (n=820),[27] GFR was found to be an independent predictor of Hb (p<0.0001). Associations between Hb and GFR were continuously significant (p<0.05) at lower levels of GFR <70 vs GFR 80–100. Hb was significantly lower in all male and female patients with GFR <70 (both p<0.0001). GFR of more than 80 ml/min/1.73 m^2 was not significantly associated with anaemia defined as Hb ≤11 g/dl (irrespective of sex) and Hb <13 g/dl in men and Hb <12 g/dl in women. (**Level 3**)

Diabetes status and estimated GFR (eGFR) (ml/min/1.73m^2) categories <30, 30–59, and 60–89 were significantly associated with an increased likelihood of anaemia, defined as Hb <12.0 g/dl for men and post-menopausal women (older than 50 years old) and Hb <11.0 for pre-menopausal women (50 years old or younger) using eGFR ≥90 as the reference.[30] (**Level 3**)

In the same study,[30] when eGFR was divided into 10 ml/min/1.73m^2 strata, the prevalence of anaemia by diabetes status was statistically significant at each of the categories between 31 and 60 ml/min/1.73m^2, but did not differ for any other categories.

In addition, in men with diabetes, significantly lower Hb levels were observed at all eGFR categories <60 ml/min/1.73m^2, whereas among women with diabetes and all study participants without diabetes (both men and women), significantly lower Hb levels were not apparent until more advanced levels of kidney impairment were observed (eGFR <31 ml/min/1.73m^2). (**Level 3**)

▷ Hb levels associated with different CCr levels in diabetic patients

Type 2 diabetic patients with mild renal impairment (CCr 60–90 ml/min/1.73 m^2)[28] were approximately twice as likely to have anaemia as diabetic patients with normal renal function, defined as Hb <130 g/l in men and Hb <120 g/l in women (CCr >90 ml/min/1.73 m^2) (p value not reported by the authors). (**Level 3**)

4.2.4 From evidence to recommendations

The comparison of diabetic and non-diabetic populations was based on a clinical perception that the diabetic population was at risk of developing anaemia of CKD at an earlier stage. The GDG felt that this perception had arisen partly because of the selected patient populations in many of the studies, the cross-sectional nature of the studies, and the lack of standardisation of estimates of renal function used in the various studies.

The current clinical perception of the GDG is that although there was a correlation between diabetes and the anaemia of CKD, the prevalence of anaemia in those with diabetes appeared greater than those without at higher levels of GFR. Within whole population studies there were similar mean haemoglobin levels between those with diabetes and those without diabetes across a range of GFRs.

It was agreed that setting a threshold value of eGFR of 60 ml/min/1.73m^2 (the boundary between stage 2 and stage 3 CKD) would be of use in helping clinicians decide whether to consider anaemia of CKD as a cause of the anaemia, although there were some concerns about whether the error around a single measurement would make this a suitable recommendation.

It was felt there was some merit in an empirical statement that supported setting an eGFR of <60 ml/min/1.73m^2 which should alert a clinician to consider anaemia of CKD as the cause, and that other causes were likely in patients with a eGFR > 60.

RECOMMENDATION

R2   An estimated glomerular filtration rate (eGFR) of <60 ml/min/1.73m^2 should trigger investigation into whether anaemia is due to CKD. When the eGFR is ≥60 ml/min/1.73m^2 the anaemia is more likely to be related to other causes.   (D)

See 3.2.1 for the associated algorithm.

4.3   Diagnostic tests to determine iron status

4.3.1   Clinical introduction

The purpose of the evidence review in this section was to identify the best combination of tests to determine iron status in patients with CKD.

The aim of determining iron status is to identify which patients need iron supplementation, as well as those who do not. Although absolute iron deficiency may occur in patients with chronic kidney disease we more frequently identify what is termed 'functional iron deficiency'. Although iron stores may seem adequate when measured by conventional indices of iron status, there may be a lack of 'freely available iron' for effective erythropoiesis in the bone marrow.

There is a lack of well-accepted gold standard tests for determining iron deficiency in the setting of CKD. While bone marrow iron stores are often regarded as the best indicator of iron status, this is not universally accepted and taking a bone marrow sample is invasive, relatively time consuming and expensive. The frequent coexisting inflammatory or infective problems in patients with CKD can complicate the interpretation of iron status parameters. For example, serum ferritin is a good marker of storage iron and decreases in iron deficiency states. However, it is also an acute phase reactant, which means it is frequently raised in inflammatory conditions, such as CKD, regardless of the iron status. All the available tests of iron status are subject to similar limitations and detailed discussion is beyond the scope of this guideline. The British Committee for Standards in Haematology is producing a document 'Evaluation of iron status', which will deal comprehensively with these issues (although not specifically in the setting of CKD). It is accepted that no single parameter can determine iron status.

In patients without CKD normal serum ferritin levels are over 20 µg/l, but in those with CKD a value of 100 µg/l is considered to be the lower limit of normal to allow for the associated mild inflammatory state. The percentage of hypochromic red cells (HRC) directly reflects the number of red blood cells with suboptimal levels of haemoglobin content (<28 g/dl) and may be determined using certain analysers. HRC <2.5% is normal and HRC >10% indicates definite iron deficiency. Measurement must be on a fresh sample (<4 hours after the blood is withdrawn) because of storage artefact. Reticulocyte haemoglobin content (CHr) may also be measured by certain analysers and is derived from the simultaneous measurement of volume and haemoglobin concentration in reticulocytes. Levels indicating functional iron deficiency depend on the analyser used. Transferrin saturation (TSAT) is a derived value and may be calculated from serum iron × 100 ÷ total iron binding capacity; or serum iron (mg /dL) × 70.9 ÷ serum transferrin (mg/dl). Transferrin levels are also influenced by inflammation and nutrition (correlating with serum albumin levels). A TSAT of <20% suggests iron deficiency.

4.3.2 Methodological introduction

A literature search identified studies which addressed the ability of tests to detect iron deficiency[60–62] and the ability of tests to predict the response to intravenous iron supplementation in patients with predefined iron parameters receiving epoetin.[63–68]

Of the six studies looking at the response to intravenous iron, five studies predefined the patient population to whom iron was given as being iron deficient (see Table 4.16). In one study[66] the response to intravenous iron was used to define the prior iron status. No study addressed the issue of loading with iron prior to epoetin administration.

Table 4.16 Definition of detection of iron deficiency		
Reference	Iron dosing regimen	Definition of positive response to iron administration, ie iron-deficient
64	1g infusion (over 2 hours)	Erythropoietic response to the iron treatment; a sustained increase in corrected reticulocyte index of one base point (ie from 1.7% to 2.7%) within 2 weeks
65	500mg to 1g infusion (over 1 hour)	>5% increase in Hct, 4 weeks after administration
66	~1g over 8 weeks	Hb response ≥15% of baseline value
67	240mg iron colloid over 2 weeks	Not reported
68	1.5g over 41.7 weeks	• Reduction in weekly epoetin dose of at least 30 U/kg/week in the subsequent 12 weeks while maintaining a target Hct of 30 to 33% • Reduction in weekly epoetin dose of at least 60 U/kg/week in the subsequent 12 weeks while maintaining a target Hct of 30 to 33%
63	1g over 10 HD treatments	• ≥5% increase in Hct or a decrease in epoetin dose if the Hct increased to more than 38%
HD = Haemodialysis.		

4.3.3 Evidence statements

▷ Studies where iron was administered

A variety of studies looked at the utility of a number of markers of iron status as indicators of iron deficiency following iron administration. Response to iron administration was variably defined by an increase in haemoglobin level and/or reduction in erythropoietin dose.

Table 4.17 Studies where iron was given

Reference	N (range)	Iron test (cut-off range in studies)	Test cut-off value	Sensitivity	Test cut-off value	Specificity	Evidence hierarchy
64–66,68	32–136	Serum ferritin (50 to 400 µg/l)	<50 µg/l	19.6%	<100 µg/l	30–78.4%	DSII[64–66] DSIII[68]
			<100 µg/l	35.3–71.4%	<50 µg/l	94.6%	
64,66	32 and 51	%HRC (>4% to >10%)	>4%	86.3%	>4%	78.4%	DSII[64,66]
			>10%	42.8 and 45.1%	>10%	80 and 100%	
64–68	32–136	TSAT (<12% to <28%)	<20%	57.1–74%	<20%	36–80%	DSII[64–67] DSIII[68]
65,66	17 and 51	Serum ferritin (<100µg/l) and TSAT (<20%)	Serum ferritin <100µg/l and TSAT <20%	33% and 68.6%	Serum ferritin (<100µg/l) and %TSAT (<20%)	67% and 60.8%	DSII[65,66]
64,66,67	32–94	Ret Hb (<26 pg to <32.5 pg)	<26 pg	100%	<26 pg	80%	DSII[64,66,67]
			<32.5 pg	23.1%	<32.5 pg	66.7%	
66	51	ZPP (>52 and >90 µmol/mol haem)	>52 µmol/mol haem	80.6%	>52 µmol/mol haem	68.7%	DSII
			>90 µmol/mol haem	13.9%	>90 µmol/mol haem	96.9%	

continued

Table 4.17 Studies where iron was given – *continued*							
Reference	N (range)	Iron test (cut-off range in studies)	Test cut-off value	Sensitivity	Test cut-off value	Specificity	Evidence hierarchy
66	51	%HRC (>6%) and other tests	%HRC >6% and Ret Hb ≤29 pg	86.3%	%HRC >6% and Ret Hb ≤29 pg	93.2%	DSII
			%HRC >6% and serum ferritin <50 ng/ml	82.4%	%HRC >6% and serum ferritin <50 ng/ml	89.2%	
			%HRC >6% and TSAT <19%	96.1%	%HRC >6% and TSAT <19%	74.3%	
			%HRC >6% and ZPP >52 mmol/ mol haem	94.9%	%HRC >6% and ZPP >52 mmol/ mol haem	71.9%	
			%HRC >6% and STR >1.5 mg/ 100 ml	85.7%	%HRC >6% and STR >1.5 mg/100 ml	73.2%	

HRC = hypochromic red cells; TSAT = transferrin saturation; Ret Hb = reticulocyte haemoglobin content; ZPP = erythrocyte zinc protoporphyrin; STR = serum transferrin receptor; PPV = positive predictive value; NPV = negative predictive value.

▷   No iron administration

Table 4.18 Studies where iron was not given

Reference	N (range)	Iron test cut-off range in studies)	Test cut-off value	Sensitivity	Test cut-off value	Specificity	Evidence hierarchy
62	63	STR (1.39 µg/ml to 3.5 µg/ml)	STR 1.39 µg/ml	84%	STR 1.39 µg/ml	30%	DSIb
			STR 3.5 µg/ml	38%	STR 3.5 µg/ml	90%	
60	25	Bone marrow examination (BME) vs other tests	BME vs Serum ferritin <200 µg/l	41%	BME vs Serum ferritin <200 µg/l	100%	DSIb
			BME vs TSAT <20%	88%	BME vs TSAT <20%	63%	
61	36	TSAT vs other tests	TSAT <15% vs Ret Hb <26 pg	73	TSAT <15% vs Ret Hb <26 pg	100	DSII
			TSAT <15% vs %HRC >2.5%	91	TSAT <15% vs %HRC >2.5%	54	
			TSAT <15% vs %HRC >5%	91	TSAT <15% vs %HRC >5%	62	

4.3.4   From evidence to recommendations

The group compared the tests based on the sensitivity, specificity and receiver operator characteristics. The group did not use the negative or positive predictive values as they were considered sensitive to demographics and epidemiology and therefore not generalisable.

These iron supplementation studies have dealt with iron deficiency or 'functional iron deficiency' (where storage iron may be adequate, but iron utilisation in red cell production is defective). The studies have not addressed the issues of whether iron supplementation could be beneficial in patients having erythropoietin even with apparently normal iron status, or when iron supplementation should be stopped because of a risk of iron overload.

Recticulocyte Hb content and the percentage of hypochromic red cells were also discussed. Neither of these tests are widely available and both are currently under a commercial patent. With respect to recticulocyte Hb content, the GDG felt that although this looked like a sensitive test, the cut-off for this test was a Hb content of less than 26pg. This was considered very low as the normal range is reported to be 31–33pg. The GDG noted that the percentage of hypochromic red cells provided the best sensitivity and specificity from a single test.

In general, the GDG noted that tests for serum ferritin and transferrin saturation were the most widely used but that they had poor sensitivity and specificity. The GDG took note, however, that these tests were both cheap and widely available. It was noted that serum ferritin was the only test addressing iron storage while the other tests reviewed in the evidence assessed iron utilisation. The GDG agreed that no single test was adequate to determine iron status. Serum ferritin showed the best correlation with bone marrow iron scores. Iron deficiency should be ascertained by a combination of serum ferritin (storage iron) and tests of iron utilisation (reticulocyte haemoglobin content, percentage of hypochromic red cells, transferrin saturation, ZPP).

RECOMMENDATIONS

R3   Serum ferritin levels may be used to assess iron deficiency in people with CKD. Because serum ferritin is an acute phase reactant and frequently raised in CKD, the diagnostic cut-off value should be interpreted differently to non-CKD patients.   (A(DS))

R4   Iron deficiency anaemia should be:
- diagnosed in people with stage 5 CKD with a ferritin level of less than 100 µg/l
- considered in people with stage 3 and 4 CKD if the ferritin level is less than 100 µg/l.   (D(GPP))

R5   In people with CKD who have serum ferritin levels greater than 100 µg/l, functional iron deficiency (and hence those patients who are most likely to benefit from intravenous iron therapy) should be defined by:
- percentage of hypochromic red cells >6%, where the test is available or
- transferrin saturation <20%, when the measurement of the percentage of hypochromic red cells is unavailable.   (B(DS))

See 3.2.1 for the associated algorithm.

4.4   Measurement of erythropoietin

4.4.1   Clinical introduction

Although anaemia in CKD may develop in response to a wide variety of causes, erythropoeitin (EPO) deficiency is the primary cause of renal anaemia. Predominantly produced by peritubular cells in the kidney, EPO is the hormone responsible for maintaining the proliferation and differentiation of erythroid progenitor cells in the bone marrow. Loss of peritubular cells leads to an inappropriately low level of circulating EPO in the face of anaemia (Figure 4.2).

We know that anaemia develops early in the course of chronic kidney disease. NHANES III found lower levels of kidney function to be associated with lower haemoglobin levels and a higher prevalence and severity of anaemia.[55] The prevalence of anaemia, defined as haemoglobin levels of less than 12 g/dl in men and less than 11 g/dl in women, increased from 1% at an estimated GFR of 60 ml/min per 1.73 m^2, to 9 and 33% at estimated GFRs of 30 and 15 ml/min per 1.73 m^2 respectively. Using the same definition of anaemia, it is suggested that in people with diabetes and CKD the prevalence of anaemia in stage 2 and 3 CKD is greater than in those without diabetes.[30] In a study of 5,380 participants from the Kidney Early Evaluation

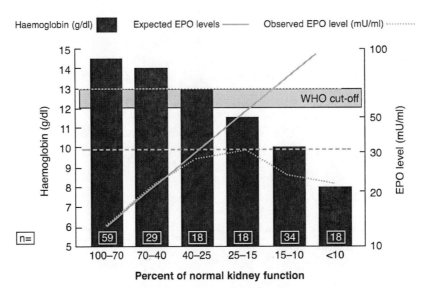

Figure 4.2 **Evolution of anaemia in CKD** (reproduced with kind permission of Dr Anatole Besarab). EPO = erythropoietin; WHO = World Health Organization.

Program, 22% of those with CKD stage 3 and diabetes had anaemia, compared with 7.9% of those with stage 3 CKD alone (p<0.001). In stage 2 CKD 7.5% of those with diabetes were anaemic compared with 5.0% of those without diabetes (p=0.015). In people with diabetes the prevalence of anaemia at all levels of GFR is greater with increasing levels of albuminuria.[28]

When patients with diabetes and CKD are stratified into those more likely to be iron-replete (TSAT>16%) and those less likely to be iron-replete (TSAT<16%) anaemia is associated with a relative lack of EPO response in those with TSAT>16%.[29]

In patients with less advanced CKD there may be some uncertainty about whether or not the anaemia is associated with lack of EPO, and this may be particularly so in transplanted patients in whom immunosuppression may also play a role in suppressing the bone marrow response. In these patients, knowledge of serum EPO levels may be beneficial and the evidence review in this section seeks to address this.

4.4.2   Methodological introduction

One cohort study,[70] six cross-sectional studies[26,29,71–74] and two longitudinal studies, prospective[75] and retrospective,[76] which examined the association between serum erythropoeitin with Hb levels or renal function, were identified in a literature search.

Notable aspects of the evidence base were:

- The studies comprised selected and unselected participants.
- Of the three studies conducted in people with diabetes, the study populations consisted of people with Type 2 diabetes without nephropathy,[76] selected people with Type 1 diabetes with diabetic nephropathy in the absence of advanced renal failure,[26] people with Type 1 and 2 diabetes.[29]
- Other causes of anaemia were explicitly ruled out in some studies.[26,70,72,75,76]

- Where reported, anaemia was defined as <13 g/l for men and <11.5 g/l for women,[76] Hb ≤11.5 g/dl for women and 12.0 g/dl for men,[26] Hb <11 g/dl,[72] Hb <12 g/dl for women and Hb <13 g/dl for men.[29]

A comprehensive literature search did not identify any studies that were suitable to address the economic aspects, therefore no health economic evidence statements are given.

4.4.3 Evidence statements

▷ Adults with diabetes

In people with Type 2 diabetes **without** nephropathy (n=62) a significant negative correlation between serum EPO and Hb levels was found (r^2=0.612, p=0.01).[76] (**Level 3**)

In contrast to the above finding, a study in people with Type 1 diabetes **with** diabetic nephropathy (in the absence of advanced renal failure) (n=27), found no significant EPO response to lower Hb levels.[26] (**Level 3**)

A cross-sectional study conducted in people with diabetes[29] found no significant EPO response in anaemic patients (defined as Hb <12 g/dl for women and Hb <13 g/dl for men) with GFR >60 ml/min/1.73m^2 or >90 ml/min/1.73m^2. (**Level 3**)

In a subgroup of iron replete diabetic patients (transferrin saturation level >16%), from the above study,[29] serum EPO levels did not change significantly with Hb level as shown below.

Table 4.19 Characteristics in anaemia and raised or normal serum EPO (Level 3)			
	No anaemia, n=554	Anaemia + normal EPO, n=131	Anaemia + raised EPO, n=37
Erythropoietin (IU/l)	15 ± 8	16 ± 7	74 ± 112*#
Haemoglobin (g/dl)	14.1 ± 1.1	11.6 ± 1.0*	11.0 ± 1.1*#
GFR (ml/min/1.73m^2)	79 ± 26	57 ± 28*	66 ± 28*#
TSAT <16%	15%	31%*	73%*#

* Vs no anaemia p<0.05. # Vs anaemia with normal levels of EPO.

▷ Children with chronic renal failure

No significant correlation was found between serum EPO and Hb/Hct levels in three studies conducted in children with chronic renal failure (n=7;[71] n=10;[74] n=37[75]). (**Level 3**)

Likewise, no significant correlation was found between serum EPO levels and renal function assessed by means of eGFR (n=37)[75] or serum creatinine (SCr) (n=30)[73] in children with chronic renal failure. (**Level 3**)

The results of a study which investigated Hb and serum EPO levels in children with chronic renal failure and healthy children are shown in Table 4.20.

Table 4.20 Hb and serum EPO in children (Level 3)			
	N	Hb (g/dl)	Mean serum EPO (U/l)
Predialysis	30	10.7 ± 2.5	36.2 (range 7 to 235)
Post-transplant	15	11.6 ± 2.6	39.5 (range 10 to 125)
Healthy children	20	13.2 ± 0.8	35.2 (range 18 to 64)

▷ Adults with chronic renal failure on conservative therapy

In patients with CKD of varying renal function (CCr 2 to 90 ml/min/1.73m^2 (n=117)), mean serum EPO levels were significantly elevated in all patients when compared with healthy controls (n=59) (p<0.01). In a subgroup analysis of patients with CCr 2–40 ml/min/1.73m^2 (n=88), CCr and serum EPO showed a positive correlation (r=0.27, p<0.015).[70] (Level 2+)

▷ Unselected population of adults

In a random sample of patients investigated by coronary angiography (n=395) stratified by renal function, a significant inverse relationship was found between serum EPO and Hb levels in participants with CCr >40 ml/min (r=-0.35, p<0.0001). No significant correlation was found, however, in participants with CCr <40 ml/min.[72] (Level 3)

4.4.4 From evidence to recommendations

Anaemia is associated with increased EPO levels in individuals without evidence of CKD but the anaemia associated with CKD is characterised by a relative lack of EPO response. However, in the clinical situation routine measurement of EPO levels is of limited value in assessing anaemia.

The GDG reached consensus on a threshold GFR of 40 ml/min, below which anaemia is most likely to be of renal aetiology and measurement of erythropoietin levels will not be required except in exceptional circumstances. At GFR levels between 40 and 60 ml/min, the utility of testing is uncertain from the existing evidence, and a research recommendation is given.

RECOMMENDATION

R6   Measurement of erythropoietin levels for the diagnosis or management of anaemia
should not be routinely considered for people with anaemia of CKD.   (D(GPP))

5 | Management of anaemia

5.1 Initiation of ESA therapy in iron-deficient patients

5.1.1 Clinical introduction

Iron management forms an essential part of the treatment of anaemia associated with CKD and availability of iron is of key importance for iron optimal erythropoiesis. Before erythropoietin treatment was available, patients with anaemia associated with CKD frequently received blood transfusions. One of the consequences of this was the progressive accumulation of iron, manifested by extremely high ferritin levels in excess of 1,500 to 5,000 µg/l. With the advent of ESA therapy this accumulated iron was rapidly mobilised, and serum ferritin levels fell accordingly. We now recognise that in order to manage the anaemia optimally, there needs to be an appropriate balance between stimulation of erythropoiesis and provision of iron as a key substrate in the manufacture of haemoglobin.

In health, iron is almost completely recycled and losses are of the order of 1 mg/day, requiring minimal replacement. Iron deficiency is the most common cause of anaemia worldwide. This is due to either negative iron balance through blood loss (commonly gastrointestinal or menstrual), or to inadequate intake (which may be nutritional or related to poor gastrointestinal absorption). Patients with CKD are particularly susceptible to gastrointestinal blood loss and additional sources of significant blood loss include routine (and non-routine) blood sampling, and blood loss on haemodialysis which may represent the need for up to an extra 3,000 mg iron per year. In the first 3 months of ESA therapy it is estimated that a haemodialysis patient needs an extra 1,000 mg of supplemental iron, underlining the importance of adequate availability of iron for optimal erythropoiesis.[77]

5.1.2 Clinical methodological introduction

A comprehensive literature search did not identify any studies that were suitable to address the clinical aspects of this section, therefore no evidence statements are given.

5.1.3 Health economics methodological introduction

One study met methodological criteria.[78] This Canadian study estimated annual cost savings of intravenous iron dextran from reductions in EPO and oral iron in patients who did not tolerate or did not respond adequately to oral iron in a 6-month prospective study with an initial goal serum ferritin of 100–200 µg/l. If an increase in haemoglobin was not achieved, transferrin saturation was measured and when less than 20%, the goal serum ferritin was increased to 200–300 µg/l. EPO was used to maintain haemoglobin levels of 9.5–10.5 g/l only if ferritin targets were met.[78]

5.1.4 Health economic evidence statements

The study found that intravenous iron dextran saved approximately Canadian $63 per patient ($3,016 total) from EPO savings and oral iron savings in 50 patients. However, the initial cost of i.v. iron dextran loading was $3,426 in the first year. Therefore, the loading dose of i.v. iron dextran offset the cost reduction in EPO and oral iron in the first year but would not apply in subsequent years. Intravenous iron dextran costs were $29,692 (Canadian $, 1996) per year in the 50 patients in the study with $30,120 of EPO savings per year and $2,738 from oral iron savings per year.[78]

5.1.5 From evidence to recommendations

There is little evidence in this area but the GDG agreed that ESAs alone should not be administered to patients with iron deficiency (ferritin level <100 µg/l). The GDG debated whether ESAs should be administered together with iron supplements. It was noted that some patients with higher GFR had a good response to iron treatment alone but that there was no evidence to support a threshold for iron stores required prior to commencing ESAs, except in patients with iron deficiency.

RECOMMENDATIONS

R7   ESA therapy should not be initiated in the presence of absolute iron deficiency without also managing the iron deficiency.   (D(GPP))

R8   In people with functional iron deficiency, iron supplements should be given concurrently when initiating ESA therapy.   (D(GPP))

Also see recommendation R40 in section 6.12.5.

5.2 Maximum iron levels in patients with anaemia of CKD

5.2.1 Clinical introduction

Iron is crucial for survival and is necessary for erythropoiesis and the production of usable energy through oxidative phosphorylation. However, iron-overload states are harmful and the potent oxidising ability of non-transferrin bound iron makes it potentially toxic. The majority of iron not actively circulating as haemoglobin is safely sequestered in the form of ferritin and hemosiderin in macrophages of the reticuloendothelial system. Molecules that hold iron tend to be very large, containing a central core of iron with a proteinaceous envelope that insulates the body from the iron atom. We know that in iron-overload states, such as haemochromatosis, in which serum ferritin levels can increase to more than 10,000 µg/l, the body is presented with unmanageable levels of free iron leading to iron-related toxicity. The focus of debate about potential iron toxicity in patients with anaemia associated with CKD revolves around the possible increased susceptibility to infectious complications and increased cardiovascular morbidity and mortality engendered by iron administration. In vitro, iron preparations enhance bacterial growth, induce leukocyte dysfunction, inhibit phagocytosis, produce reactive oxygen species, increase oxidative stress, consume antioxidants and, at very high doses, promote lipid peroxidation and cell death. These observations have led to concern that too much iron might translate these in vitro phenomena into adverse infectious and cardiovascular in vivo effects.

5.2.2 Methodological introduction

A comprehensive literature search did not identify any studies that were suitable to address the clinical or economic aspects of this section, therefore no evidence statements are given.

5.2.3 From evidence to recommendations

Because of the lack of evidence, it was agreed that an upper limit of 800 µg/l of ferritin should be used in line with the current European Best Practice Guidelines.* This level is drawn from data on iron toxicity studies performed in the pre-ESA era that demonstrated that high ferritin levels >1,000 µg/l led to the deposition of iron in tissues. However, in practice, in order to prevent serum ferritin from rising above 800 µg/l a patient's iron dose should be reviewed if their serum ferritin levels exceed 500 µg/l. It was noted that it was not known whether there are any long-term consequences related to the administration of intravenous iron as this route bypassed normal absorption routes and homeostatic mechanisms.

It should be noted that ferritin is an acute phase protein that is increased during inflammatory events, this affects the interpretation of some of the studies reviewed.

RECOMMENDATION

R9   In people treated with iron, serum ferritin levels should not rise above 800 µg/l. In order to prevent this, the dose of iron should be reviewed when serum ferritin levels reach 500 µg/l.   (D (GPP))

5.3 Clinical utility of ESA therapy in iron-replete patients

5.3.1 Clinical introduction

Patients who are iron replete (ferritin >100 µg/l and %HRC <6% or TSAT ≥20%) yet still have anaemia associated with CKD will not achieve target haemoglobin levels without administration of ESAs. Should all patients regardless of the clinical situation and their functional status receive ESAs? Estimates of the number of people in England and Wales with significant CKD (eGFR <60 ml/min) and a haemoglobin level below 11 g/dl not currently receiving ESAs suggest that the potential number requiring anaemia management is 108,000. However, this estimate was made from an unselected population that will have included those with causes of anaemia other than CKD. A significant number may not have been iron replete, and the mean age of the cohort was 75.1 ± 11.63 years. The National Service Framework for Older People states that 'NHS services will be provided, regardless of age, on the basis of clinical need alone'. For many older patients improvement in quality of life is their paramount need, and older people should not necessarily be excluded from these treatments. Becoming able to move around your house independently and therefore not needing admission to a care home would clearly be a successful outcome in treating anaemia.

---

* At the time of writing the current European guidelines were: European best practice guidelines for the management of anemia in patients with chronic renal failure. *Nephrology Dialysis Transplantation* 1999;14(Suppl 5):1–50.

The key goals in the management of anaemia are increased exercise capacity, improved quality of life, improved cognitive function, improved sexual function, reduced transfusion requirements, regression/prevention of left ventricular hypertrophy, improved morbidity, prevention of progression of renal disease, reduced risk of hospitalisation, and reduced mortality. We do not yet have the evidence that all of these goals are achievable and there may be certain patients whose physical and mental status renders these goals unachievable from the outset. Clearly these patients will not therefore benefit from administration of ESAs.

5.3.2 Methodological introduction

A comprehensive literature search did not identify any studies that were suitable to address the clinical or economic aspects of this section, therefore no evidence statements are given.

5.3.3 From evidence to recommendations

The GDG expected there to be a paucity of literature in this area. The reason for investigating the evidence base in this section was to determine whether there were any subgroups of patients in whom the administration of ESAs may be of little clinical benefit.

The GDG discussed whether they considered there were any patient subgroups with a Hb level below 11 g/dl and with stage 3–5 CKD who should not be considered for treatment with ESAs. The GDG felt that it was a matter of clinical judgement, based on a patient's individual circumstances (eg presence of comorbidities), as to whether a patient would benefit from the administration of ESAs.

The GDG considered it important to note that antibody mediated pure red cell aplasia (PRCA) does occur sporadically and this was one group of patients where epoetin administration should be very carefully considered.

The GDG felt the most relevant issue was how to best focus resources in the wider CKD population to provide the most benefit. The lack of evidence would suggest this is an area where research is required. The GDG discussed that where there is uncertainty over the benefits a patient may gain from ESA therapy, a trial of ESA therapy and assessment of response may be indicated prior to continuing long-term treatment. The GDG felt that the patient was a good judge of whether the treatment had any noticeable improvement on their quality of life and did not feel there was any need to recommend any formal tests. The GDG felt strongly that the decision to actively manage an individual patient's anaemia should be made by an experienced clinician, but that this did not necessarily have to be a renal physician.

RECOMMENDATIONS

R10   The pros and cons of a trial of anaemia management should be discussed between the clinician, the person with anaemia of CKD and their families and carers if applicable. (D (GPP))

R11   ESAs need not be administered where the presence of comorbidities, or the prognosis, is likely to negate the benefits of correcting the anaemia. (D (GPP))

R12   A trial of anaemia correction should be initiated when there is uncertainty over whether the presence of comorbidities, or the prognosis, would negate benefit from correcting the anaemia with ESAs.   **(D (GPP))**

R13   Where a trial of ESA therapy has been performed, the effectiveness of the trial should be assessed after an agreed interval. Where appropriate, a mutual decision should be agreed between the clinician, the person with anaemia of CKD and their families and carers on whether or not to continue ESA therapy.   **(D (GPP))**

R14   All people started on ESA therapy should be reviewed after an agreed interval in order to decide whether or not to continue using ESAs.   **(D(GPP))**

5.4   Nutritional supplements

5.4.1   Clinical introduction

Vitamins are essential cofactors that regulate the metabolic pathways from which lipids, proteins and carbohydrates are generated and processed. The uraemic environment is responsible for the development of significant alterations in serum levels, body stores and functions of many vitamins.

In patients with more advanced CKD (stages 4 and 5) the dietary restrictions imposed for potassium and phosphate inevitably limit the intake of some vitamins from natural sources. More recently dietary counselling has focused more on nutritional support than dietary restrictions, with people eating more liberal diets to try and optimise nutritional status. Currently there are no recommendations or guidance as to which population would benefit from vitamin supplementation and in what quantity. Much of our information about supplementation of vitamins comes from studies with small subject numbers, over short periods of time. Many of the studies only address vitamin requirements in the dialysis-dependent population, excluding predialysis patients.

Reasons to support vitamin supplementation include dietary restrictions, uraemic toxins, drug–nutrient interactions and the dialysis process itself. Water soluble vitamins are lost during both haemodialysis (HD) and continuous ambulatory peritoneal dialysis (CAPD). However, this may be offset by the altered kinetics caused by renal failure which may result in reduced urinary losses or renal catabolism. The fact that CKD affects the normal absorption, retention and activity of the necessary micronutrients which support all aspects of carbohydrate, protein and lipid metabolism, further strengthens the evidence in favour of supplementation.

Less is known about the nutritional requirements of fat soluble vitamins in patients with CKD. Studies report anything from subnormal through normal to enhanced levels. In practice supplementation with fat soluble vitamins is not recommended.

Data remain incomplete on individual requirements of vitamins, the handling of vitamins in uraemia, the vitamin status of uraemic patients and the effect of vitamin administration.

Carnitine is synthesised in the body from two essential amino acids, lysine and methionine, whereas glutathione is a peptide containing the amino acids glutamic acid, cysteine and glycine. Carnitine and glutathione have both been implicated in enhancing responsiveness to EPO in CKD patients but there are few studies to date. In practice, this is not done routinely.

Although much is known about the prevalence of macronutrient deficiency in renal patients, nutritional status in CKD is beyond the scope of this guideline. This section focuses on micronutrient supplementation and its effect on the treatment of anaemia due to CKD.

5.4.2 Methodological introduction

A comprehensive literature search identified eight studies. Of these, two studies addressed vitamin C: a cross-over RCT[79] and a non-randomised controlled trial.[80] One RCT addressed folic acid.[81] Five studies addressed carnitine supplementation, which consisted of three RCTs,[82–84] a cross-over RCT[85] and a before and after study.[86]

Eleven studies had methodological limitations and were thus excluded from the evidence statements. These include four which addressed vitamin C,[87–90] one which addressed vitamin E,[91] one which addressed folate,[92] and five which addressed carnitine supplementation.[93–97]

Notable aspects of the evidence base were:
- No studies addressing vitamin E or glutathione were found.
- The meta-analysis investigating carnitine supplementation[93] did not meet quality criteria, hence the studies within it[82–84] were individually appraised.
- One study was conducted in children.[86]
- One study[79] was conducted in a pre-selected patient population.

A comprehensive literature search did not identify any studies that were suitable to address the economic aspects of this section.

5.4.3 Evidence statements

▷ Vitamin C

Haemodialysis patients

A non-randomised trial (n=52)[80] where 100 mg ascorbic acid was administered i.v. three times weekly in one group (n=23) and as an adjunct to ESA and i.v. iron in another, found no significant change in Hb levels from baseline in either group after 6 months. In addition, no changes were identified in either group in any of the eight domains of quality of life assessed using the Short-Form 36 (SF 36) scale. (**Level 2+**)

In a randomised controlled trial (RCT) of cross-over design (n=27),[79] where ascorbic acid 1,500 mg/week was administered i.v. for 3 months, Hb increased ($p<0.01$ in group I and $p<0.005$ in group II) and TSAT increased (both group I and group II $p<0.001$), whereas ferritin decreased ($p<0.004$ in group I and $p<0.001$ in group II) when compared with baseline levels. Epoetin doses, however, remained unchanged in both groups. (**Level 1+**)

▷ Folic acid

Haemodialysis patients

Reticulocyte counts (both $p<0.05$) and Hct levels (both $p<0.01$) increased from baseline levels in both sets of patients receiving folic acid 5 mg three times a week over 12 months (n=10) and patients whose folic acid supplementation had been stopped over this time period (n=10). Hct levels increased further (both p<0.01) in the 6-month follow-up period after folic acid supplementation had been stopped in both groups of patients. There were no differences, however, in response to epoetin between the two groups.[81] (**Level 1+**)

▷ Carnitine

Haemodialysis patients

No differences were observed in any of the five domains of quality of life as assessed by the Kidney Disease Questionnaire or in overall quality of life, in a RCT of cross-over design (n=16) in which placebo or 20 mg/kg L-carnitine were administered i.v. over a 12-week period. Similarly, no differences were observed in epoetin dose or Hb levels.[85] (**Level 1+**)

No differences were observed in epoetin dose requirement or Hct and reticulocyte counts in a 6-month study investigating the effects of supplementation with 1 g L-carnitine three times a week in elderly patients (n=28), after which patients were followed up for 3 months.[82] (**Level 1+**)

No differences were found when patients treated with epoetin were supplemented with 1 g carnitine three times a week or placebo (n=24) for 6 months and compared in terms of epoetin dose, endogenous epoetin levels or Hct and iron levels.[83] (**Level 1+**)

No significant changes in epoetin dose requirement were observed between patients supplemented with either 5 mg/kg (n=15) or 25 mg/kg (n=5) L-carnitine vs placebo (n=20) over 8 months. However, a greater reduction in change in epoetin dose was observed in the carnitine treated group (p<0.05) and a higher epoetin resistance index (epoetin dose:Hb ratio) (p<0.02). Additionally, after 4 months, there were significant negative correlations between plasma free carnitine, plasma total carnitine and plasma free carnitine:plasma total carnitine to EPO dose and ERI in both treatment groups.[84] (**Level 1+**)

Paediatric haemodialysis and peritoneal dialysis patients

Total carnitine and free carnitine increased significantly from baseline (both p <0.05) after 26 weeks treatment with orally administered L-carnitine 20 mg/kg daily in both haemodialysis (n=8) and peritoneal dialysis patients (n=4), with a mean age of 10.2 years. Acylcarnitine increased only in haemodialysis patients (n=8) after 26 weeks. Despite this, no changes were observed in Hb levels or epoetin dose from baseline in both sets of patients. In addition, no correlation was found between epoetin dose or Hb levels with total carnitine, free carnitine and acylcarnitine levels.[86] (**Level 3**)

5.4.4 From evidence to recommendations

It was concluded that there was no evidence to support the adjunctive use of vitamin C, folic acid or carnitine supplements in the treatment of anaemia of CKD. There was very little evidence available for the CKD population and no evidence in the predialysis population. It was considered acceptable to extrapolate the conclusions to the predialysis population.

With regard to vitamin C, the appraised studies administered very high doses (1,500 mg/wk, 1,000 mg/wk and 100 mg/wk). A dose of 50 mg/week was considered to be a more appropriate supplement given in clinical practice to renal patients. The biological basis for the administration of vitamin C was related to aiding the mobilisation of iron and promoting effective erythropoiesis. The evidence base was small.

In clinical practice, when patients are given folate supplements this is generally for other reasons than the correction of anaemia. The studies appraised on carnitine supplementation gave negative results.

RECOMMENDATION

R15   Supplements of vitamin C, folic acid or carnitine should not be prescribed as adjuvants specifically for the treatment of anaemia of CKD.   (A)

5.5   Androgens

5.5.1   Clinical introduction

Interest in the use of androgens as adjunctive treatment in the management of anaemia associated with CKD stems from their use prior to the availability of ESAs. A number of early studies[98–102] suggested a beneficial effect on renal anaemia by treatment with androgens, although notably one double blind cross-over trial of nandrolone decanoate failed to show a sustained significant effect on haemoglobin level or red cell mass.[103] However, their regular use was abandoned because of the requirement for parenteral administration and a number of adverse effects such as acne, flushing of skin, hirsutism, changes in voice, masculinisation, amenorrhoea and increasing libido, together with adverse effects related to liver function such as peliosis as well as hepatocellular adenoma and carcinoma.

The mechanism of action of androgens on erythropoiesis is still not completely understood and mechanisms proposed include increased production of endogenous erythropoietin, synergism with ESAs, enhanced sensitivity of erythroid precursors to erythropoietin, increased red cell survival, and a direct effect on erythroid precursors. There is thus a potential role for androgens in enhancing the effectiveness and reducing the dose requirements of available ESAs.

5.5.2   Methodological introduction

A literature search identified eight studies, including two RCTs,[104,105] three cohort studies[106–108] and one before and after study.[109]

Two studies[110,111] had methodological limitations and were therefore excluded from the evidence statements.

The GDG agreed that the following outcomes were priorities:
- mortality and morbidity
- improved response to ESAs
- quality of life
- Hb/Hct level
- ESA dose
- adverse effects.

Notable aspects of the evidence base were:
- The studies were investigating:
  – epoetin vs nandrolone[104,107]
  – epoetin vs epoetin and nandrolone[105,106]

- epoetin and nandrolone (no control group)[109]
- Nandrolone alone (no control group).[108]
- Although side effects were noted in some studies,[105,108,109] the authors did not attempt to quantify all of these.
- The studies were conducted in both male and female patients except for two studies, [104,106] which were conducted solely in male patients.

5.5.3 Evidence statements

▷ Hb/Hct levels

Haemodialysis patients

In a before and after study conducted in male (n=9) and female (n=8) patients,[109] Hb (p=0.001) and Hct (p=0.003) levels increased following adjuvant therapy with epoetin (3,000 U/week s.c.) and nandrolone decanoate (100 mg i.m. weekly) for 6 months. When stratified into sex of patients, Hb and Hct levels (both p=0.01) were higher only in female patients. (**Level 3**)

In a cohort study conducted in male (n=67) and female (n=17) patients,[108] Hb and Hct levels rose (both p<0.01) following 6 months' therapy with nandrolone decanoate 200 mg i.m. weekly. Although baseline Hb levels were higher in the male patients (p<0.05), the increase with respect to baseline levels was similar in both sexes throughout the study. In order to evaluate the influence of other factors, patients were divided into the following:

- non-responders (Hb increase <1 g/dl with respect to baseline; n=28)
- mild responders (Hb increase 1–1.9 g/dl with respect to baseline; n=18)
- good responders (Hb increase 2–2.9 g/dl with respect to baseline; n=25)
- excellent responders (Hb increase >2.9 g/dl with respect to baseline; n=13).

Only age was significantly associated with response to androgen therapy (p<0.01). When the cohort was stratified into ages less than 46 years (n=29), 46–55 years (n=28) and more than 55 years (n=27), only the latter two groups showed improvement in Hb levels (both p<0.01) following androgen therapy. (**Level 2+**)

A 6-month cohort study conducted to compare the effect of 200 mg nandrolone decanoate i.m. once weekly in male patients aged over 50 years (n=18) vs epoetin 6,000 IU a week in male and female patients aged less than 50 years (n=22) found an increase in Hb levels in both groups (both p<0.01), despite a drop in serum ferritin levels in the epoetin treatment group (p<0.01).[107] (**Level 2+**)

In a cohort study[106] conducted over 12 weeks in male patients treated with epoetin 6,000 U i.v. 3 times a week (n=7) vs epoetin 6,000 U i.v. 3 times a week and 100 mg nandrolone decanoate i.m. once a week (n=8), Hct values increased in the group receiving adjuvant therapy (p<0.001) after 12 weeks and no transfusions were required in either group. (**Level 2+**)

A RCT conducted in predominantly black male and female patients administered with epoetin 4,500 U per week vs epoetin 4,500 U per week (n=10; 4 men and 6 women) and nandrolone 100 mg i.m. once a week (n=9; 7 men and 2 women) over 26 weeks found a significant increase in Hct in both treatment groups when compared with baseline values (p=0.003 and p=0.001 respectively). However, the rise in Hct was greater in the epoetin plus androgen group (p=0.012) when compared with epoetin alone.[105] (**Level 1+**)

CAPD patients

Hb and Hct levels increased in both treatment groups in a RCT[104] investigating influence of epoetin initiated at 50 U/kg/week and tailored to target Hb of 11–13 g/dl vs nandrolone 200 mg i.m. once weekly (both p<0.001) when compared with baseline values. However, these increases in Hb and Hct levels were not significantly different when the treatment groups were compared with each other. (**Level 1+**)

▷ Epoetin dose

Haemodialysis patients

In a before and after study conducted in male (n=9) and female (n=8) patients,[109] weekly epoetin doses following adjuvant therapy with nandrolone decanoate (100 mg i.m. weekly for 6 months) did not change significantly, either in the overall cohort or when stratified into male and female patients. (**Level 3**)

In a cohort study conducted over 12 weeks in male patients treated with epoetin (6,000 U i.v. three times a week) (n=7) vs epoetin (6,000 U i.v. three times a week) and nandrolone decanoate 100 mg i.m. once a week (n=8), no difference was observed in epoetin dose between the two treatment groups.[106] (**Level 2+**)

▷ Adverse events—serum triglycerides

Haemodialysis patients

In a cohort study conducted in male (n=67) and female (n=17) patients, serum triglycerides increased (p<0.01) after therapy with nandrolone decanoate 200 mg i.m. weekly for 6 months.[108] (**Level 2+**)

A 6-month cohort study conducted to compare the effect of nandrolone decanoate (200 mg i.m. once weekly) in male patients aged over 50 years (n=18) vs epoetin (6,000 IU a week) in male and female patients aged less than 50 years (n=22) found an increase in serum triglycerides in the androgen group (p<0.001).[107] (**Level 2+**)

5.5.4 From evidence to recommendations

The rationale for the administration of androgens to patients with anaemia of CKD was historical in that androgens were administered in the pre-ESA era. The studies had administered nandrolone decanoate but this androgen is no longer used in clinical practice. The doses of nandrolone administered in the studies were considered to be supraphysiological. The group agreed that there was some evidence of efficacy in that the administration of androgens could reduce the dose of ESA required but were concerned about the potential side effects and considered this an outdated approach to anaemia management.

RECOMMENDATION

R16   In people with anaemia of CKD, androgens should not be used to treat the anaemia.   (C)

5.6 Hyperparathyroidism

5.6.1 Clinical introduction

Elevations in serum parathyroid hormone (PTH) concentration (secondary hyperparathyroidism) are seen early in CKD and are common when the estimated GFR is <60 ml/min (stage 3 CKD onwards).[112–114] Elevation of PTH in the stage 3 and 4 CKD populations predicts the development of more severe hyperparathyroidism, which in turn is clearly associated with increased skeletal and cardiovascular morbidity and mortality.[115] Whether hyperparathyroidism causes anaemia and resistance to treatment of anaemia, and if it does, what degree of hyperparathyroidism is clinically important, remain controversial. Potential mechanisms include a direct effect of PTH on endogenous erythropoietin synthesis, on bone marrow erythroid progenitors, and on red cell survival through accelerated haemolysis, and an indirect effect through induction of bone marrow fibrosis. This section looks at whether treatment of hyperparathyroidism in people with anaemia associated with CKD improves the management of anaemia in terms of haemoglobin level achieved and dose of ESA required, and also attempts to determine when treatment should be considered.

5.6.2 Methodological introduction

A literature search identified seven studies. These consisted of a cohort study,[116] a two-part study comprising a cohort study and prospective before and after study,[117] a two-part study comprising a prospective longitudinal study and cohort study,[118] a prospective before and after study and cohort study,[119] a prospective longitudinal study,[120] and two retrospective before and after studies.[121,122]

Six studies[123–128] had methodological limitations and were therefore excluded from the evidence statements.

The GDG agreed that the following outcomes were priorities:
- parathyroid hormone levels
- mortality and morbidity
- quality of life
- ESA dose
- improved response to ESA
- plasma erythropoietin levels
- reduction in ESA resistance
- Hb/Hct level.

Notable aspects of the evidence base were:
- Treatment for parathyroidism was stratified into drug-based with calcitriol,[117,118] alfacalcidol,[120] or surgery.[116,117,121,122]

A comprehensive literature search did not identify any studies that were suitable to address the economic aspects of this section, therefore no health economic evidence statements are given.

5.6.3 Evidence statements

Table 5.1 Summary of evidence for appraised studies

Reference	Drug-based therapy	Sample size	Baseline iPTH levels (pg/ml)	Treatment duration	Outcome	Effect	Level of evidence
117	Calcitriol 2 µg	n=16	778 ± 172.7	6 months	n=7 responders iPTH Hct Epoetin dose	↓ ↑ ↓	Level 2+
120	Alfacalcidol 6 mg	n=12	~475	18 months	iPTH Hb	↓ ↑	Level 3
118	Calcitriol i.v. 2 µg	n=28	811.6 ± 327	12 months	Hb/Hct IPTH	↑ ↓	Level 3
118	Calcitriol i.v. 2 µg	n=28	811.6 ± 327	12 months	Epoetin use (n=21) vs No Epoetin (n=7) Epoetin dose	No change	Level 2+
118	Calcitriol i.v. 2 µg	n=28	811.6 ± 327	12 months	Responders (n=19) vs non-responders (n=9) Hct Epoetin dose	↑ No change	Level 2+

Author/ Study ID	Surgical procedure	Sample size	Basal iPTH levels (pg/ml)	Length of follow-up after surgery	Outcome	Effect	Level of evidence
122	Subtotal parathyroidectomy (n=9) and total parathyroidectomy with forearm autotransplantation (n=1)	n=10	Not reported	6 months	iPTH Hct Epoetin dose	↓ ↑ ↓	Level 3
117	Total parathyroidectomy with forearm autotransplantation	n=3	976 ± 436.1	6 months	iPTH Hct Epoetin dose	↓ ↑ ↓	Level 3+
121	Subtotal parathyroidectomy	n=19	1,726 ± 1,347	1–2 years (n=44)	Hb	No change	Level 3
	Total parathyroidectomy and autotransplantation	n=10	913 ± 380	3–5 years (n=24)	Hb	↑	
	Total parathyroidectomy	n=10	1,006 ± 668				
	Partial parathyroidectomy (removal of 2–3 parathyroid glands)	n=6	1,176 ± 3346				

continued

Table 5.1 Summary of evidence for appraised studies – *continued*

Author/ Study ID	Surgical procedure	Sample size	Basal iPTH levels (pg/ml)	Length of follow-up after surgery	Outcome	Effect	Level of evidence
119	Total parathyroidectomy and forearm autotransplantation	n=29 Note n=7 underwent reoperation for recurrences in neck and forearm	873 ± 710.8	12 months	iPTH Hb Plasma erythropoietin	↓ ↑ ↑	Level 3
				12 months	Epoetin use (n=23) vs No Epoetin (n=6) Epoetin dose	No change	Level 2+
116	Total parathyroidectomy and forearm autotransplantation	n=32 1,338 ± 350.6	Responders	3 months	n=17 responders (≥10% Hb increase post-PTX) vs	No change	Level 2+
			Non-responders 1,228 ± 290.8		n=15 non-responders	No change No difference	
					Hb Serum erythropoietin	↓ but no difference between the 2 groups	
					iPTH		

↑ = significant increase; ↓ = significant decrease; PTX = parathyroidectomy.

5.6.4   From evidence to recommendations

Treatment of hyperparathyroidism secondary to CKD is part of good clinical practice as is routine monitoring of PTH levels in patients with CKD. Early control of hyperparathyroidism is crucial for preventing metabolic bone disease and treating hyperparathyroidism is beneficial to anaemia management. The strategies used do not differ in patients with CKD whether they are anaemic or not. On the evidence available, it was not felt to be appropriate to recommend specific interventions and the British,[129] American[130] and European[131] treatment guidelines in the management of renal osteodystrophy which are aimed at attainment of target PTH, calcium and phosphate concentrations should be followed.

RECOMMENDATION

R17   In people with anaemia of CKD, clinically relevant hyperparathyroidism should be treated to improve the management of the anaemia.   (C)

5.7   Patient-centred care: ESAs

5.7.1   Clinical introduction

The ESAs currently available in clinical practice differ in terms of frequency of administration and route of administration. The ESAs currently available in clinical practice may be administered either subcutaneously or intravenously. Darbepoetin is likely to require less frequent administration than the erythropoietins, while the erythropoietins are likely to require less frequent administration and a lower dose when administered subcutaneously vs intravenously. Logistically it is easier for patients not on haemodialysis to receive ESAs subcutaneously by self-administration or administration by their carer/practice nurse at home; patients on haemodialysis may also elect to receive their ESA either through self-administration or from dialysis staff at the end of haemodialysis.

Key considerations for patients with anaemia associated with kidney disease are that:

- ESAs are prescribed when clinically indicated.
- The ESA supply, route of supply and storage arrangements are clearly defined, secure and convenient.
- The administration and monitoring of anaemia treatment is as efficient, comfortable and least disruptive as possible.

5.7.2   Methodological introduction

Seven studies were identified, including two RCTs,[132,133] one of which was of cross-over design,[133] one retrospective longitudinal study,[134] one retrospective case series,[135] and three cross-sectional studies.[136–138]

One study[139] had methodological limitations and was thus excluded from the evidence statements. The buffer used in the preparation in the cross-over study[133] is no longer used, and the paper was therefore not considered further.

Notable aspects of the evidence base were:

- The studies conducted using questionnaires were limited by the use of closed questions in their design,[134,136,138] with the exception of one study,[137] which reported the use of both closed and open questions.
- All the studies using questionnaires were cross-sectional, with the exception of one study,[134] which was of longitudinal design.

A comprehensive literature search did not identify any studies that were suitable to address the economic aspects of this section, therefore no evidence statements are given.

5.7.3 Evidence statements

▷ Route of administration – effect on quality of life

Haemodialysis patients

In a 24-week cross-over study[132] where s.c. was compared with i.v. administration, quality of life assessed by means of the Kidney Disease Questionnaire (KDQ), which consists of five domains, found improvements from epoetin administration (both intravenous and subcutaneous) in the physical ($p<0.05$) and fatigue ($p<0.05$) domains, but no significant differences between the two modes of administration in any other domains.[133] (**Level 1+**)

▷ Adherence and ESA administration

Peritoneal dialysis patients

In a retrospective longitudinal study,[134] 19 of 54 (35%) patients administering s.c. epoetin in the home setting were non-concordant (defined as less than 90% of the prescribed dose used), with the most commonly reported reason being forgetfulness. Missing dialysis exchanges, completion of secondary education and younger age were found to be independent predictors of non-adherence ($r^2=0.36$). (**Level 3**)

In a retrospective study,[135] 30 of 55 (55%) patients administering epoetin s.c. in the home setting were non-concordant (defined as less than 90% of the prescribed dose used). Whether another person administered the ESA on behalf of the patient was the only significant correlation with concordance ($r=0.46$, $p=0.005$). (**Level 3**)

Haemodialysis and continuous ambulatory and automated peritoneal dialysis patients

In a cross-sectional study,[136] concordance ranged from 24–33%, with the over-60 age group least likely to miss an epoetin dose and reduced frequency of administration associated with less missed doses. The majority of patients were likely to self-administer. Fewer injections were preferred by 72.5%, with the under-60 age group preferring once-weekly because of convenience, pain on injection and epoetin storage. (**Level 3**)

Predialysis, hospital and home haemodialysis and continuous ambulatory peritoneal dialysis patients

In a cross-sectional study,[137] 57 of 86 (66%) patients reported they never missed doses, while 31% admitted to occasionally missing doses and 3% admitted to frequently missing doses. Following a missed dose, the majority (39%) informed the renal unit, 27% carried on as usual after the missed dose, 19% administered the missed dose as soon as they remembered. The majority (55%) of patients preferred self-administration of epoetin, with 17% reporting difficulties with injection preparation and 17% reporting pain at the injection site. (**Level 3**)

▷ Communication and obtaining of ESA

Predialysis, hospital and home haemodialysis and continuous ambulatory peritoneal dialysis patients

In a cross-sectional study,[137] the majority of patients (89%) reported the renal unit anaemia nurse to be the preferred source of information. However, most patients (59%) reported they did not need more information. Most requests for information were found to be about how epoetin works (31%), possible side effects (29%) and what epoetin is for (26%). Epoetin supply was found to be mostly by GPs (71%), although 20 patients (23%) reported that their GPs had refused to supply epoetin. Most patients preferred obtaining epoetin supplies from a community pharmacy (n=63). (**Level 3**)

Predialysis, dialysis and transplant patients

In a cross-sectional study,[138] most (91%) anaemic patients received epoetin therapy. Of the 4% that were refused epoetin, the reasons given were that the GP could not pay for it (50%) and that the hospital could not pay for it (20%). (**Level 3**)

▷ EPO administration – effect on quality of life

Predialysis, dialysis and transplant patients

In a cross-sectional study,[138] sleep disturbance, tiredness and ability to attend a 9am to 5pm job were found to be associated with baseline Hb and post-treatment levels. Patients whose post-treatment Hb levels had increased from below 11 g/dl to above 11 g/dl were 1.8 times more likely to report an improvement in QoL. Patients with post-treatment Hb levels >11 g/dl were 1.9 times more likely to agree with the statement 'I can attend a 9am–5pm job'. (**Level 3**)

5.7.4 From evidence to recommendations

The evidence from seven studies contained outcome data on quality of life, pain, concordance, obtaining ESAs and communication with patients.

The data supported the view that patient preferences and experiences should be taken into account, where possible, when decisions are reached about treatment with ESAs. The patient should be given access to sufficient information about their condition and its treatment to allow them to make informed choices about the management of their condition (for example, whether to have supervised- or self-administration of ESAs). It was noted that some studies had shown an increased lack of concordance in some groups who had chosen self-administration.[134,135] Patients need to be aware of the consequences of poor concordance and one study highlighted that a reduced frequency of administration of ESAs resulted in increased concordance.[136] Currently many patients have difficulties securing a supply of ESAs. Many patients are unable to obtain ESAs from their local hospital or GP practice and have the ESAs delivered to them at home. This can cause problems in finding the capacity to refrigerate large quantities of drugs. This area needs to be addressed by healthcare providers to ensure adequate drug supply and storage facilities for patients.

RECOMMENDATIONS

R18   People offered ESA therapy, and their GPs, should be given information about why
ESA therapy is required, how it works, and what benefits and side effects may be
experienced.   (D)

R19   When managing the treatment of people with anaemia of CKD, there should be agreed
protocols defining roles and responsibilities of healthcare professionals in primary and
secondary care.   (D(GPP))

R20   People receiving ESA therapy should be informed about the importance of concordance
with therapy and the consequences of poor concordance.   (D)

R21   When prescribing ESA therapy, healthcare professionals should take into account patient
preferences about supervised- or self-administration, dose frequency, pain on injection,
method of supplying ESA and storage.   (D(GPP))

R22   In order for people to self-administer their ESA in a way that is clinically effective and
safe, arrangements should be made to provide ready, reasonable and uninterrupted
access to supplies.   (D)

5.8   Patient education programmes

5.8.1   Clinical introduction

Patient self-management is one of the cornerstones of chronic disease management, enabling
patients some degree of control of their own disease process. The level of independence each
individual achieves depends as much on the quality of the information and self-management
tools provided as it does on the ability of the individual patient. Patient education programmes
are therefore of paramount importance in achieving effective patient self-management.

Structured patient education involves planned education that covers all aspects of anaemia
management and is flexible in content, is relevant to a person's clinical and psychological needs,
and is adaptable to their educational and cultural background. A well-planned education
course will provide a written outline, be delivered by trained educators (preferably someone
who is both well versed in the principles of patient education and is competent to teach the
programme), be quality assured, and provide the opportunity for feedback.

5.8.2   Methodological introduction

A comprehensive literature search did not identify any clinical or health economic studies that
were suitable to address this section.

5.8.3   From evidence to recommendations

Patient education was considered to be hugely important and information should be available
at different levels. Adequate information helps patients to make decisions about their treatment
and illness, although it was noted that there might be some patients who will wish to remain
passive about their condition.

Patient education should meet the individual needs of each patient and five themes drawn from recent work in the area[140] were considered to be important:

- practical management of anaemia
- knowledge (about symptoms, iron and ESA management and product delivery and storage)
- professional support (contact information, community services, continuity of care, monitoring, feedback on progress of results)
- lifestyle (diet, physical exercise, maintaining normality, meeting other patients)
- adaptation (causes of anaemia, associated medications, phases of treatment, previous information and expectations, resolution of symptoms).

RECOMMENDATION

R23   Culturally and age-appropriate patient education programmes should be offered to all people diagnosed with anaemia of CKD and their families and carers. These should be repeated as requested, and according to the changing circumstances of the patient. They should include the following key areas:

- practical information about how anaemia of CKD is managed
- knowledge (eg about symptoms, iron management, causes of anaemia, associated medications, phases of treatment)
- professional support (eg contact information, community services, continuity of care, monitoring, feedback on progress of results)
- lifestyle (eg diet, physical exercise, maintaining normality, meeting other patients)
- adaptation to chronic disease (eg previous information and expectations, resolution of symptoms). (D(GPP))

6 | Assessment and optimisation of erythropoiesis

6.1 Benefits of treatment with ESAs

6.1.1 Clinical introduction

The introduction of ESAs into clinical practice nearly 20 years ago dramatically changed the management of anaemia associated with chronic kidney disease. Prior to ESA therapy, dialysis-dependent patients were profoundly anaemic, frequently manifesting haemoglobin levels of between 6 and 7 g/dl, the only treatments available being blood transfusions, iron or androgen therapy. The potential benefits associated with anaemia treatment are numerous. These include avoidance of blood transfusions with their attendant risks of sensitisation against future transplantation, iron overload, blood-borne disease and transfusion reactions; improved quality of life and physical functioning; improved cognitive and sexual function; cardiovascular benefits in terms of structure, function, incidence and prevalence of disease; and reduced hospitalisation, morbidity and mortality.

6.1.2 Clinical methodological introduction

Four studies were identified. A meta-analysis (epoetin vs placebo or no treatment),[141] two multisite RCTs (epoetin vs placebo),[142,143] one cohort study (epoetin vs no treatment)[144] and a retrospective longitudinal study.[145] Two studies[145,146] had methodological limitations and were therefore excluded.

The outcomes to assess the efficacy of the ESA preparations in comparison with placebo or no treatment were morbidity, left ventricular hypertrophy, left ventricular function, mortality, hospitalisation and dialysis adequacy.

Notable aspects of the evidence base:
- All studies except for two included in the meta-analysis[141] did not explicitly state if they used epoetin-alfa or epoetin-beta.
- The study durations ranged from 12 weeks to 3.5 years.
- Studies included in the meta-analysis[141] achieved a lower Hb level and excluded patients with significant comorbidities.
- In one study[143] red cell transfusions were given to placebo or treatment arms when required.

6.1.3 Clinical evidence statements

▷ Quality of life

Predialysis patients

Of the studies in the meta-analysis,[141] Kleinman (1989), by means of a visual analogue scale rating of three questions, found an improvement in quality of life after 12 weeks with a mean difference of 35 (95% CI 12.47 to 57.53). Roth (1994), by means of the Sickness Impact Profile and other validated tests, found an improvement at 48 weeks, with the control group having decreased physical function (p=0.03) and the epoetin group having increased physical function (p=0.015) as well as increased energy (p=0.045). However, the number of domains assessed in this study was not provided by the authors. (**Level 1+**)

Haemodialysis patients

In one study[142] an improvement in four out of five categories of the Kidney Disease Questionnaire were found (physical p<0.001; fatigue p<0.001; relationships p=0.001; depression p=0.018). In addition, the Sickness Impact Profile questionnaire found an improvement in quality of life as reflected by the reduction of the global scores (p=0.024) and the physical scores (p=0.005). Psychosocial scores did not change significantly. (**Level 1+**)

▷ Mortality

There were insufficient mortality data available from the meta-analysis[141] and the RCT[143] to write evidence statements.

▷ Hospitalisation

Study participants new haemodialysis patients

No statistically significant difference in hospitalisation between epoetin and placebo treatment groups was found, including when stratified and analysed into admission type, age group and history of cardiovascular disease.[144] (**Level 2+**)

6.1.4 Health economics methodological introduction

Three studies were identified.[14,147,148] One study[149] did not meet met quality criteria and therefore no evidence statements were made.

One study contained a cost-effectiveness analysis before and during epoetin therapy.[14] It was predominantly a cost-savings analysis with 1990 to 1991 UK£ and earlier costs. However, the 1990 to 1991 or earlier cost data meant that there was insufficient data from which to derive evidence statements for application to the current NHS context.

One study compared cost per QALY results in five European countries including the UK.[147] This study used QALYs as the effectiveness measure. Nevertheless, costs were derived from 1988 values, which indicates there are insufficient data from which to derive evidence statements for the current NHS context.

An additional study[148] evaluated the cost per QALY of epoetin using the same framework as the Leese study[147] (1988 values), but updated data with values from the year 2000 in the UK.

6.1.5 Health economics evidence statements

The cost per QALY of ESA therapy in the UK using data from the year 2000 was £17,067. The model was most sensitive to changes in the QALY gain. The baseline QALY gain used to derive the cost per QALY was 0.088 per year. However, if a 0.17 QALY gain occurs, the cost per QALY drops to £8,809, conversely if a 0.02 QALY gain occurred, the cost per QALY would increase to £74,876.[148]

6.1.6 From evidence to recommendations

One study[141] was appraised that assessed mortality but the GDG considered the study to be underpowered to determine whether there was a clinically important difference in mortality rate. The GDG felt that the evidence was not sufficient to make a sound evidence statement.

The GDG concluded that the study of people receiving peritoneal dialysis[143] did not contribute meaningful data as the study duration was too short (12 weeks) to assess mortality.

Of the outcomes assessed, the GDG felt there was only good evidence supporting improvement in quality of life through ESA therapy. The GDG noted that the studies had small sample sizes and had concerns over the statistical validity of the evidence. The studies in the meta-analysis[141] achieved a low target haemoglobin and the patients that may have shown the greatest benefits were excluded from the studies.

The GDG noted that because highly selected populations were included in these studies, the effects reported were not as large as those observed in the unselected patient populations observed in clinical practice.

The GDG concluded on the basis of qualitative data and clinical experience that ESAs are of value.

Health economic evidence was presented to the group. The GDG agreed that one study was presented that was sufficiently robust to be included and gave useful cost per QALY information in the UK context.[148] However, as the model was sensitive to the gain in QALY, the GDG felt further economic evidence is required before definitive statements about the cost effectiveness are made. The GDG felt the other studies:

- estimated the price but underestimated the benefit of the treatment (n=24)[147]
- were based on a study design that could introduce bias,[149] or
- were based on historical cost data that no longer had relevance to the current NHS context.[14]

RECOMMENDATION

R24 Treatment with ESAs should be offered to people with anaemia of CKD who are likely to benefit in terms of quality of life and physical function.   (A)

See 3.2.2 for the associated algorithm.

6.2 Blood transfusions

6.2.1 Clinical introduction

The potential risks of blood transfusion include transfusion reactions, immunomodulation, iron overload and transfusion transmitted infections.

Data concerning adverse transfusion events in the UK are collected by the Serious Hazards of Transfusion (SHOT) group. Their 2003 report included data from 351/415 UK hospitals (see **www.shotuk.org**). Since the inception of SHOT in 1996 there has been an increase in the number of adverse transfusion incidents reported with now over 2,000 recorded in the SHOT database (Table 6.1). Although the numbers of transfusion-transmitted infections reported are low, the list of infections that may be potentially transmitted is growing rapidly and includes hepatitis B, C and G, human immunodeficiency virus (HIV), human t-lymphocytotrophic virus (HTLV-1), transfusion transmitted virus (TTV), cytomegalovirus (CMV), Creutzfeld-Jakob disease (CJD), human herpes virus (HHV-8), leishmaniasis, Lyme disease, malaria, babesiosis and toxoplasmosis.

Table 6.1 Serious Hazards of Transfusion (SHOT) Report 2003

SHOT category	Reported cases 1996–2003, n (%)	Risk category	Estimated risk
Incorrect blood component transfused	1393 (66.7)	Risk of incorrect blood component transfused	1 in 16,500
Acute transfusion reaction	233 (11.2)	Risk of ABO incompatibility	1 in 102,200
Delayed transfusion reaction	213 (10.2)		
Transfusion-related acute lung injury	139 (6.7)	Risk of transfusion-related acute lung injury	1 in 165,000
Transfusion-transmitted infection	45 (2.2)		
Post-transfusion purpura	44 (2.1)	Risk of serious hazard	1 in 11,000
Transfusion-associated GVHD	13 (0.6)	Risk of major morbidity	1 in 92,000
Unclassified	7 (0.3)	Risk of death	1 in 255,500

Prior to the introduction of ESAs, in addition to the immediate risks of transfusion reactions and infection, the two biggest concerns for patients with CKD were sensitisation against future transplantation and iron overload. This was complicated by the evidence suggesting that transfusion prior to transplantation may actually be beneficial in terms of future transplant outcome. This had been first suggested in 1973.[150] However, a subsequent assessment following the introduction of ciclosporin failed to confirm a benefit[151] and this subject remains controversial. Donor-specific transfusion prior to living-related transplantation appears favourable[152] but in cadaveric transplantation the picture is less clear. A multicentre randomised controlled trial of transfusion of three units of packed cells demonstrated improved graft survival at 1 and 5 years.[153] However, approximately 5% of the patients in this study became sensitised, and had not been transplanted by the end of the study period. In children, a retrospective study hinted at a beneficial effect from transfusion of 1–5 units of blood, but this beneficial effect was lost with greater numbers of units transfused.[154] A recent study looking at the causes of sensitisation of potential renal allograft recipients in Ireland in the post-EPO era demonstrated that the level of sensitisation clearly increased with the number of units transfused.[155] Non-sensitised participants (PRA <10%) received a mean of 5.65 units

(SEM 1.38), sensitised participants (PRA 11–59%) a mean of 9.8 units (SEM 3.17), significantly sensitised (PRA 60–79%) a mean of 18.2 units (SEM 6.51), while highly sensitised participants (PRA ≥80%) received a mean of 37.8 units (SEM 8.4). There was a direct relationship between the waiting time for transplantation and the degree of sensitisation.

Although blood transfusion is not the only factor related to recipient sensitisation, since ESAs have become more freely available and the use of routine blood transfusion for correction of anaemia has disappeared, sensitisation has markedly reduced (Figure 6.1).

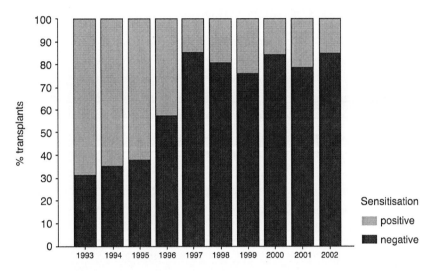

Figure 6.1 Recipient pre-transplant HLA-specific sensitisation: adult recipients of cadaver donor kidneys (Manchester Kidney Transplants, NWKTA Audit Project, January 2003)

6.2.2 Methodological introduction

A comprehensive literature search identified two studies, a case-control study[156] and a before and after study.[157]

Five studies[155,158–161] had methodological limitations and were therefore excluded from the evidence statements.

A comprehensive literature search did not identify any studies that were suitable to address the economic aspects of this section, therefore no health economic evidence statements are given.

6.2.3 Evidence statements

▷ Immunological parameters / sensitisation

Haemodialysis patients

No significant differences were observed in the analyses of lymphocytes, monocytes, T8, T4, T11, T13, Ia and B1 cells or T4/T8 ratios in patients who had previously received five or more transfusions over 6 months (n=30) when compared with a matched lightly transfused group (n=30).[156] (**Level 2+**)

Dialysis patients

More patients in the lightly transfused group developed narrowly reactive antibodies (reacting with 10–29% panel cells) in comparison with the more heavily transfused group who developed antibodies against ≥30% panel cells. Sensitisation increased waiting time for transplants both in subsequently transplanted patients (p<0.003) and the entire patient population regardless of transplantation (p<0.03).[157] (**Level 3**)

6.2.4 From evidence to recommendations

The GDG noted the lack of evidence on important factors that would impact on the risks of correcting anaemia with regular blood transfusions, such as blood borne viruses and iron overload. In the late 1970s and early 1980s there was evidence that giving blood transfusions before transplantation improved transplant outcome and most units had a deliberate transfusion policy; most research focused on the risks of sensitisation which meant that certain donors would be excluded if the antibodies were directed to their lymphocytes (detected in the 'cross match test'). Around the mid-1980s transmission of blood borne viruses by transfusion (in particular HIV) became a major public health issue. At the same time ciclosporin came into regular use. Ciclosporin improved survival, and taken together with the risk of the transmission of blood borne viruses and the availability of erythropoietin for treating anaemia, deliberate transfusion was discontinued.

The GDG considered the evidence on the immunological risks of correcting anaemia with regular blood transfusions. They agreed that the evidence relating to the development of cytotoxic antibodies to lymphocytes[157] was more clinically relevant than the data on the levels of different subtypes of lymphocytes induced by transfusion.[156] It was noted that blood transfusion increased the percentage of cytotoxic antibodies in dialysis patients resulting in not only an increased waiting time for a transplant but also increased difficulty in finding a cross match negative donor.

The GDG felt it was important to stress the benefits of transfusion when clinically indicated for blood loss or in some cases the correction of anaemia (eg in some elderly patients). The GDG agreed that there were general clinical reasons to avoid blood transfusion and the relevant haematology guidelines should be followed (eg the British Committee for Standards in Haematology (BCSH) guidelines **www.bcshguidelines.com**).

RECOMMENDATIONS

R25   In people with anaemia of CKD, in whom kidney transplant is a treatment option, blood transfusions should be avoided where possible.   (**D**)

R26   In people with anaemia of CKD there may be situations where a transfusion is indicated clinically. In these cases, the relevant haematology guidelines[162] should be followed.   (**D (GPP)**)

6.3 Comparison of ESAs

6.3.1 Clinical introduction

Erythropoiesis stimulating agents (ESAs) are agents stimulating production of red blood cells through a direct or indirect action on erythropoietin receptors of erythroid progenitor cells in the bone marrow. There are three licensed forms of ESA currently available in England and Wales,[*] two short-acting (epoetin alfa and epoetin beta) and one long-acting (Darbepoetin alfa).

Epoetin alfa is a glycoprotein manufactured by recombinant DNA technology and has the same biological effects as endogenous erythropoietin. It has an apparent molecular weight of 32,000 to 40,000 daltons and is produced by mammalian cells into which the human erythropoietin gene has been introduced. The protein fraction of the molecule contributes about 58% and consists of 165 amino acids. Four carbohydrate chains are attached via three N-glycosidic bonds and one O-glycosidic bond to the protein moiety. Epoetin alfa obtained by gene technology is identical in its amino acid and carbohydrate composition to endogenous human erythropoietin that has been isolated from the urine of anaemic patients.

In both patients and normal volunteers, after intravenous administration of epoetin alfa, serum levels decline in a monoexponential manner and the volume of distribution is similar to that of the plasma volume. The half-life in normal volunteers is approximately 5 hours, but in patients with renal failure it is prolonged to approximately 9 hours. With multiple injections of epoetin alfa, half-life and clearance decrease. Measurement of epoetin alfa following multiple dose intravenous administration revealed a half-life of approximately 4 hours in normal volunteers and approximately 5 hours in renal failure patients. A half-life of approximately 6 hours has been reported in children. After s.c. administration of epoetin alfa, peak serum levels occur between 12 and 18 hours later. The peak is always well below the peak achieved using the i.v. route (approximately 1/20th of the value). The bioavailability of subcutaneous injectable epoetin alfa is approximately 20% lower than that of the intravenous drug. Elevated levels of epoetin alfa are found in the serum 48 hours after a subcutaneous dose, but not after an intravenous dose.

Epoetin beta is also identical in its amino acid and carbohydrate composition to erythropoietin that has been isolated from the urine of anaemic patients. Pharmacokinetic investigations in healthy volunteers and uraemic patients show that the half-life of intravenously administered epoetin beta is between 4 and 12 hours and that the distribution volume corresponds to one to two times the plasma volume. After subcutaneous administration of epoetin beta to uraemic patients, the protracted absorption results in a serum concentration plateau, whereby the maximum concentration is reached after an average of 12 to 28 hours. The terminal half-life is higher than after intravenous administration, with an average of 13 to 28 hours. The bioavailability of epoetin beta after subcutaneous administration is between 23 and 42% when compared with intravenous administration.

The biological efficacy of epoetin alfa and epoetin beta has been demonstrated in various animal models in vivo (normal and anaemic rats, polycythaemic mice). After administration of

---

[*] Epoetin delta was granted marketing approval in March 2002 by EMEA and introduction into the UK market is pending. Prescribers should be aware of developments in the available products and should check the most recent Summaries of Product Characteristics.

epoetin alfa and epoetin beta, the number of erythrocytes, the Hb values and reticulocyte counts increase as well as the Fe-incorporation rate. It has been shown in cell cultures of human bone marrow cells that epoetin alfa and epoetin beta stimulate erythropoiesis specifically and do not affect leucopoiesis.

Darbepoetin alfa is an erythropoiesis stimulating protein, closely related to erythropoietin, that is produced by recombinant DNA technology. It is a 165-amino acid protein that differs from recombinant human erythropoietin in containing five N-linked oligosaccharide chains. The two additional N-glycosylation sites result from amino acid substitutions in the erythropoietin peptide backbone.

Darbepoetin stimulates erythropoiesis by the same mechanism as endogenous erythropoietin and epoetin alfa and beta. Following subcutaneous administration, absorption is slow and rate limiting. The observed half-life in patients with renal failure was 49 hours (range: 27 to 89 hours) and reflects the rate of absorption. Following intravenous administration to patients with renal failure, serum concentration-time profiles are biphasic, with a distribution half-life of approximately 1.4 hours and a mean terminal half-life of 21 hours. Following subcutaneous administration in patients with renal failure peak concentrations occur at 34 hours (range: 24 to 72 hours). Following intravenous administration, the terminal half-life of darbepoetin is approximately three times longer than epoetin alfa. The bioavailability of darbepoetin in patients with renal failure after subcutaneous administration is 37% (range: 30% to 50%).

6.3.2 Clinical methodological introduction

▷ Epoetin alfa vs epoetin beta

There were no studies comparing epoetin alfa and epoetin beta.

▷ Darbepoetin vs epoetin alfa

One multisite RCT[163] comparing darbepoetin and epoetin alfa was identified. One study[164] was excluded because of methodological limitations.

Notable aspects of the evidence base were:
- Of the 28-week study duration,[163] the first 20 weeks were a dose titration and stabilisation period.

▷ Darbepoetin vs epoetin beta

A comprehensive literature search identified one open-label RCT comparing darbepoetin and epoetin beta.[165]

Notable aspects of the evidence base were:
- Darbepoetin dose was converted at 200 IU:1 μg according to the manufacturer's dose conversion.

The GDG agreed that the following outcomes were priorities in assessing the efficacy of the ESA preparations:

- haemoglobin level
- ESA dose
- morbidity
- mortality
- quality of life
- left ventricular hypertrophy and left ventricular function.

6.3.3 Clinical evidence statements

▷ Darbepoetin vs epoetin alfa

Haemodialysis patients

Efficacy

A mean change in Hb level between baseline and evaluation periods of 0.13 g/dl (95% CI –0.08 to 0.33) was above the pre-defined margin of –1.0 g/dl and therefore implied that no significant difference was observed between the two treatment groups.[163] (**Level 1+**)

No significant difference was observed for:

- haemoglobin variability assessed as variance in haemoglobin
- percentage values within the Hb target range
- percentage values within the therapeutic range and instability of Hb levels requiring a dose change within the two treatment groups.[163] (**Level 1+**)

Dose change from baseline to evaluation was similar for both treatment groups.[163] (**Level 1+**)

The number of patients with dose changes during the titration and evaluation periods was similar for both treatment groups.[163] (**Level 1+**)

Safety

The type and frequency of adverse events was similar in both treatment groups, with no antibody formation to either treatment detected.[163] (**Level 2+**)

▷ Darbepoetin vs epoetin beta

Haemodialysis patients

Efficacy

There was no significant difference in maintaining Hb at 11–12 g/dl between darbepoetin (n=81) and epoetin beta (n=81), both administered s.c. weekly over 9 months.[165] (**Level 1+**)

Dose

Over the 9-months study duration, median dose fell in the darbepoetin arm (p=0.006), but increased in the epoetin beta arm (p=0.002). When converted into the same units (IU/kg/week) using the manufacturer's dose conversion, darbepoetin dose required to achieve the same Hb outcome was significantly lower than epoetin beta dose at 9 months (95%CI 17–61 IU/kg/week, p<0.001).[165] (**Level 1+**)

Blood pressure

Blood pressure did not change significantly in the course of the study in either treatment arm.[165] (**Level 1+**)

6.3.4 Health economics methodological introduction

Only one economic evaluation[166] was found that compared darbepoetin and epoetin alfa. However, this study had methodological limitations and therefore no evidence statements were made.[*]

6.3.5 From evidence to recommendations

The GDG agreed that the evidence statements from the multisite RCT support the summary that there is no difference between darbepoetin and epoetin alfa for the outcomes measured, in a selected group of patients who were stable.[163]

Evidence statements on efficacy suggest that both darbepoetin and epoetin beta effectively maintain target haemoglobin levels. ESAs are made available to NHS trusts through a system of tendering for local supply contracts. Costs therefore vary between locations and over time. The recommendation below outlines the considerations in agreeing on a first choice ESA rather than specifying a particular agent for all patients. This is intended to allow flexibility for local units over the lifetime of the guideline while providing useful advice in selecting the best treatment for the patient.

RECOMMENDATION

R27   The choice of ESA should be discussed with the person with anaemia of CKD when initiating treatment and at subsequent review, taking into consideration the patient's dialysis status, the route of administration and the local availability of ESAs. There is no evidence to distinguish between ESAs in terms of efficacy.   **(A)**

6.4   Early or deferred ESA therapy

6.4.1   Clinical introduction

The patients most likely to derive the greatest long-term benefit from correction of anaemia are those with chronic kidney disease who are predialysis. Early intervention to correct anaemia has the potential to impact on the progression of chronic kidney disease and affect patient morbidity,

---

[*] In interpreting economic evaluation of ESAs, it should be borne in mind that different units will have developed their own pricing structures which may differ considerably from BNF list prices.

hospitalisation rates, quality of life, and mortality. The key goals in the management of anaemia are increased exercise capacity, improved quality of life, improved cognitive function, improved sexual function, reduced transfusion requirements, regression/prevention of left ventricular hypertrophy, improved morbidity, prevention of progression of renal disease, reduced risk of hospitalisation, and reduced mortality.

6.4.2 Methodological introduction

A comprehensive literature search identified two studies.[167,168]

Notable aspects of the evidence base were:
- One study[167] was conducted in a selected patient population, recruiting only patients without diabetes.
- Target Hb levels in both studies were not met. The target Hb level for one study[167] was 13 g/dl, however, the mean Hb levels achieved was 12.9 g/dl (standard deviation 0.4) in the early treatment group and 10.3 g/dl (standard deviation 1.0) in the deferred treatment group.
- The target Hb levels for the other study[168] were 12–13 g/dl in the early treatment group and 9–10 g/dl in the deferred treatment group, while mean levels achieved were 12.1 g/dl (standard deviation 1.4) and 10.8 g/dl (standard deviation 1.3) respectively.

A comprehensive literature search did not identify any studies that were suitable to address the economic aspects of this section, therefore no health economic evidence statements are given.

6.4.3 Evidence statements

▷ Left ventricular mass index

Predialysis patients

No significant differences were observed in left ventricular mass index measurements in a 2-year study[168] conducted to maintain Hb 12–13 g/dl (n=75) vs 9–10 g/dl (n=80) using epoetin. Treatment was initiated in the latter group when Hb was <9 g/dl at two consecutive assessments 2 months apart or <8 g/dl at any one time. (**Level 1++**)

▷ Renal function

Predialysis patients

No significant differences were observed in renal function (eGFR) in a 2-year study[168] conducted to maintain Hb 12–13 g/dl (n=75) vs 9–10 g/dl (n=80) using epoetin. However, eGFR progressively decreased in the two treatment arms (p<0.001). Treatment was initiated in the latter group when Hb was <9 g/dl at two consecutive assessments 2 months apart or <8 g/dl at any one time. (**Level 1++**)

In a study conducted over 22.5 months in patients without diabetes with similar baseline creatinine clearance levels, where initiation of epoetin treatment was early (n=45) vs deferred (n=43, Hb <9 g/dl) and administered to achieve a target Hb ≥13 g/dl, the adjusted relative hazard for doubling of serum creatinine, renal replacement or death was 0.37 (95% CI 0.18 to

0.73, p=0.004) in the early epoetin treatment arm. Additionally, the risk of an event increased 2.23-fold (95% CI 1.56 to 3.18, p<0.01) per 1 mg/dl higher serum creatinine at baseline. Similarly, the adjusted relative hazard for renal replacement or death was 0.38 (95% CI 0.19 to 0.76, p=0.006) in the early epoetin treatment arm and the risk of an event increased 2.25-fold (95% CI 1.57 to 3.23, p<0.001) per 1 mg/dl higher serum creatinine at baseline.[167] (**Level 1+**)

▷ Hypertension

Predialysis patients

In a 2-year study conducted to maintain Hb 12–13 g/dl (n=75) vs 9–10 g/dl (n=80), using epoetin and initiated in the latter group when Hb was <9 g/dl at two consecutive assessments 2 months apart or <8 g/dl at any one time, no significant differences were observed in systolic and diastolic blood pressure.[168] (**Level 1++**)

In a study conducted over 22.5 months in non-diabetic patients with similar baseline creatinine clearance levels, whereby initiation of epoetin treatment was early (n=45) vs deferred (n=43, Hb <9 g/dl) and administered to achieve a target Hb ≥13 g/dl, no significant differences were observed in systolic and diastolic blood pressure between the 2 treatment arms.[167] (**Level 1+**)

▷ Quality of life

Predialysis patients

In a 2-year study conducted to maintain Hb 12–13 g/dl (n=75) vs 9–10 g/dl (n=80), using epoetin and initiated in the latter group when Hb was <9 g/dl at two consecutive assessments 2 months apart or <8 g/dl at any one time, no significant differences were observed in quality of life domains, as assessed by the Renal Quality of Life Profile and Short Form 36 (SF 36) questionnaires.[168] (**Level 1++**)

6.4.4 From evidence to recommendations

Both studies presented in the evidence were considered to be methodologically sound. The GDG felt that the study by Gouva et al[167] had achieved the study aims (in terms of level of Hb achieved) and showed a significant reduction in rate of renal progression. The study by Rogers et al[168] did not achieve the study aim and showed no significant difference in any outcome. It was not considered possible to reach any sound conclusions on the basis of these papers.

The GDG felt they could not make any recommendations on this area based on these studies alone. The evidence showed no contraindication to early correction of anaemia.

6.5 Coordinating care

6.5.1 Clinical introduction

During the past decade in the UK, the management of anaemia associated with CKD has evolved into a nurse-led programme in many renal units. The introduction of specialist nurses dedicated to managing anaemia in CKD is in response to an increased number of patients receiving treatment for renal anaemia. This role may also be undertaken by other health professionals, such as pharmacists, the goal being to deliver an effective, efficient, patient-centred anaemia service. The inefficient use of ESAs, the increase in the use of intravenous iron therapy, the requirement for patient monitoring and for regular audit have also highlighted the need to have a dedicated person responsible for anaemia management. Specialist nurses are able to work within protocols, become supplementary and extended nurse prescribers, and therefore can manage this group of patients with a high degree of independence.

The exact role of these health professionals will depend on how the anaemia management programme is set up and run, and this will vary from unit to unit. For example, they may be responsible for a small case load such as haemodialysis patients and the management may be lead by a computer algorithm or clinicians, or they may be responsible for managing the entire anaemia programme across all modalities.

6.5.2 Methodological introduction

A comprehensive literature search identified a before and after study.[169] However, because of methodological limitations, it was excluded from the evidence statements.

A comprehensive literature search did not identify any health economic studies that were suitable to address this issue.

6.5.3 From evidence to recommendations

The GDG felt that there is a benefit to having a healthcare worker identified as having responsibility for the provision of care of specific patients. There are core social and professional skills that will be needed which can be delivered by people from different clinical backgrounds, for example nurses or pharmacists. The cost effectiveness varies according to the activity of the anaemia coordinator and improves with increasingly independent activity.

RECOMMENDATION

R28   People with anaemia of CKD should have access to a designated contact person or
persons who have principal responsibility for their anaemia management and who
have skills in the following activities:

- monitoring and managing a caseload of patients in line with locally agreed protocols
- providing information, education and support to empower patients and their families and carers to participate in their care
- coordinating an anaemia service for people with CKD, working between secondary and primary care and providing a single point of contact, to ensure patients receive a seamless service of the highest standard
- prescribing medicines related to anaemia management and monitoring their effectiveness.   (D(GPP))

6.6 Providing ESAs

6.6.1 Clinical introduction

Patients with anaemia associated with CKD do not necessarily need to receive their treatment within a hospital setting. One of the core principles involved in improving health outcomes for people with long-term conditions is improved care in primary care and community settings, emphasising the patient's role in self-care and thus promoting independence and empowering patients to allow them to take control of their lives. Provision of ESA therapy is no different and can only be achieved with an appropriate infrastructure and an effective delivery system enabling the right patients to get the right ESA at the right time and in the right place.

6.6.2 Methodological introduction

A comprehensive literature search identified one cross-sectional study.[137]

A comprehensive literature search did not identify any health economic studies that were suitable to address this issue.

6.6.3 Evidence statements

Predialysis, hospital and home haemodialysis and continuous ambulatory peritoneal dialysis patients

In a cross-sectional study[137] of 87 patients, ESA supply was found to be mostly by GPs (71%), followed by hospital pharmacies (29%), although 20 patients (23%) reported that their GPs had refused to supply an ESA. Of 124 patients, 51% preferred obtaining their ESA supplies from a community pharmacy, while 19% preferred a hospital pharmacy. The reasons for both community and hospital pharmacy were primarily convenience (55%), followed by easier access (16%), supply always available (13%), shorter waiting time (10%) and provision of a larger supply (6%).

6.6.4 From evidence to recommendations

One cross-sectional study showed that there were issues for patients in obtaining ESA supplies from GPs and that many patients obtained their drugs from community pharmacists or the hospital pharmacy. This study was completed prior to the introduction of home delivery schemes run by pharmaceutical companies. However, there was often little flexibility in the day/time that companies could provide a home delivery service to patients. Hospitals source the cheapest supply of ESAs from the drug companies and cost was also an important factor in the provision of ESAs. However, every patient should have a secure supply of ESAs obtained from a source that took the patients choice and lifestyle into consideration.

It was noted that maintaining choice for patients in how ESAs are supplied and administered was vital as some patients were dependant on hospitals to administer drugs or did not have the facilities to store large quantities of drugs.

RECOMMENDATION

R29   ESA therapy should be clinically effective, consistent and safe in people with anaemia
of CKD. To achieve this, the prescriber and patient should agree a plan that is
patient-centred and includes: (D (GPP))
- continuity of drug supply
- flexibility of where the drug is delivered and administered
- the lifestyle and preferences of the patient
- cost of drug supply
- desire for self-care where appropriate
- regular review of the plan in light of changing needs.

6.7 ESAs: optimal route of administration

6.7.1 Clinical introduction

Three ESAs are currently available in the UK, two short-acting (epoetin alfa and epoetin beta)
and one long-acting (darbepoetin). Short-acting ESAs are more suited to short dose intervals
and long-acting ESAs are more suited to dosing intervals of at least a week or more. Intravenous
administration of ESAs obviously requires intravenous access and is therefore logistically
difficult in predialysis, peritoneal dialysis, and transplant patients. Patients on haemodialysis
treatment may therefore easily receive ESA therapy by any route, and at varying dose intervals,
whereas other patients with anaemia associated with CKD will normally require subcutaneous
administration with dosing intervals largely determined by the ESA used.

6.7.2 Methodological introduction

A literature search identified 58 studies. Because of the high number of retrieved studies, studies
were grouped into the various identified factors and only the studies describing clinically
relevant factors of the highest level of evidence and those which used regression analysis were
included in the evidence statements. These are detailed below:

Table 6.2 Studies included in the evidence statements	
Route of administration	**Study type**
170	RCT
171	RCT, cross-over
172	RCT
173	RCT
174	RCT, cross-over
132	RCT
175	RCT

continued

Table 6.2 Studies included in the evidence statements – *continued*	
Frequency of administration	**Study type**
176	RCT
177	RCT
178	RCT
Patient population	**Study type**
179	Non-randomised study
180	Cohort study
181	Cohort study
Hypertension	**Study type**
182	Prospective longitudinal study
Patient preference	**Study type**
183	Prospective cross-sectional cross-over study

Four studies[184–187] were excluded from the evidence statements because of methodological limitations. The buffer used in the preparation in the patient preference study is no longer used, and the paper was therefore not considered further.

The GDG agreed the following outcomes were priorities:

- mortality
- morbidity
- quality of life
- pain
- Hb/Hct levels
- complications
- patient satisfaction
- patient concordance
- patient compliance
- ESA dose required.

A comprehensive literature search found no suitable health economic studies to address this issue.

6.7.3 Evidence statements

▷ Haematocrit and arterial pressure

Haemodialysis patients

A 6-month study[182] conducted in hypertensive patients (n=13) found no significant changes in Hct after conversion of epoetin administration from the intravenous route to the subcutaneous route. However, a significant decrease in predialysis mean arterial pressure from the first month was observed (p<0.05). (**Level 3**)

▷ Antihypertensive dose requirement

Continuous ambulatory peritoneal dialysis patients

In a 16-week RCT,[173] a mean epoetin dose of 84 ± 9 U/kg/week administered subcutaneously vs a mean dose of 133 ± 7 U/kg/week administered intraperitonealy increased antihypertensive therapy in both groups, but no significant difference was found between the two groups. (**Level 1+**)

▷ Pain

Haemodialysis patients

In an RCT study[183] (n=208) comparing intravenous and subcutaneous routes for three times weekly treatment,[172] level of discomfort assessed using the Visual Analogue Scale found similar scores between the two modes of administration. (**Level 1++**)

▷ ESA dose requirement

Haemodialysis (HD) and continuous ambulatory peritoneal dialysis (CAPD) patients

In a 130-day non-randomised study investigating epoetin administration by subcutaneous vs intravenous routes (n=29),[179] the time and cumulative dose required to achieve a target Hb of 11.3 g/dl was lower in the s.c. treated HD (n=9) and CAPD groups (n=9) (both p<0.05) when compared with the i.v. treated HD group (n=11). In addition, once target Hb was achieved, a lower epoetin dose was required in the HD and CAPD subcutaneous groups (p<0.05) when compared with the intravenously treated HD group. There were no differences in epoetin dose requirement between the subcutaneously treated HD and CAPD groups. In agreement with this finding, no differences were observed in both Hb/Hct levels and epoetin requirement over 6 months in a cohort study[181] comparing epoetin administration by the subcutaneous route in CAPD (n=8) vs HD (n=7) patients. (**Level 2+**)

In contrast to the above findings, a 24-week cohort study[180] comparing HD (n=10) vs CAPD (n=11) when epoetin was administered by the subcutaneous route found that the epoetin requirements, both to achieve and to maintain a target Hct of 30%, were higher in the HD group (both p<0.05). (**Level 2+**)

▷ Frequency of administration

Haemodialysis patients

Three RCTs of 12–16 weeks duration[176–178] investigating subcutaneous epoetin administration once weekly vs twice weekly[177] and once weekly vs three times weekly,[176,178] found no significant difference in epoetin requirement or rise in Hb levels[176–177] or systolic blood pressure in both groups.[176] (**Level 1+**)

▷ Efficacy

Haemodialysis patients

Four RCTs of the following durations:

- 12 months[170]
- 8 to 24-week active treatment duration with 24-week follow-up period[132]
- 48-week duration consisting of a 26-week maintenance phase[172]
- 4-months[175]

compared subcutaneous vs intravenous epoetin administration three times weekly and found no significant differences in Hb/Hct levels between the two groups,[132,170,172,175] although time to reach the target Hb was higher in the intravenously treated group (p=0.037) of one study.[132]

One study[170] found no significant differences between the two modes of administration of epoetin in terms of the weight-standardised epoetin doses at monthly intervals or the cumulative epoetin dose to achieve target Hct 28–36%. One other study[132] found greater epoetin requirement in the intravenous group (p=0.019) during the Hb stabilisation (correction) phase of the study, but once target Hb was achieved in both groups, no difference was observed. Two other studies[172,175] found that the epoetin requirement was less for the subcutaneously treated group (p=0.02).

In addition, one study[132] assessed quality of life using the Kidney Disease Questionnaire and showed improvement in the physical and fatigue domains of both the intravenous and subcutaneous groups. These improvements, however, did not differ between the two routes of administration at any time. (**Level 1+ and 1++**)

In contrast to the above findings, in a randomised cross-over study[174] patients received similar doses of subcutaneous epoetin once (A1), twice (A2) or three times (A3) weekly (n=43), and crossed over to receiving intravenous epoetin once (B1), twice (B2) or three times (B3) weekly (n=38) over 3 months (or vice versa). A significant rise (p<0.001) in Hb was noted during the subcutaneous phase, whereas the intravenous phase was associated with a fall in Hb (p<0.001). (**Level 1++**)

Continuous ambulatory peritoneal dialysis (CAPD) patients

In a 16-week RCT (n=19), subcutaneously administered epoetin produced a rise in Hb levels (p<0.01), whereas intraperitonealy administered epoetin did not, despite a higher mean.[173] (**Level 1+**)

Peritoneal dialysis patients

Similarly to the CAPD patients, in a 32-week randomised cross-over study (n=13)[171] Hb levels in patients receiving intraperitoneal epoetin fell (p=0.03) when compared with the subcutaneous route. In support of this finding, the 16-week area under the Hct response curve (p=0.001) and the mean slope of the 16-week Hct response curve (p=0.05) were greater for subcutaneous dosing. Conversely, epoetin requirement per week was greater with intraperitoneal treatment in terms of the 16-week dose-requirement area under the curve (p=0.0029) and the slope of the 16-week dose requirement curve (p=0.017). In addition, the mean total dose per week over the entire study was greater for the intraperitoneal route (p<0.01). (**Level 1+**)

6.7.4 Health economics: cost-minimisation analysis

A meta-analysis of trial data was conducted to compare costs for subcutaneous and intravenous administration of ESAs. Only epoetin beta had sufficient data to allow a valid comparison. Subcutaneous administration appears to save £1,100 ± £727 per patient per year, compared with intravenous administration. Full details are given in Appendix D.

6.7.5 From evidence to recommendations

Of the factors addressed, hypertension was not shown to be affected by the route of administration of ESAs. The patient population, pain of injection, frequency of administration, efficacy and cost were all important factors in determining the route of administration.

The following points were also relevant:
- It was not practicable to administer ESAs by the intravenous route in patients not on haemodialysis. Equally, patients on haemodialysis may prefer to receive their ESA via the intravenous route.
- Frequency of administration was also considered important for nursing compliance. In some units it was considered better to give ESAs routinely at all dialysis visits rather than at every third.
- The half-life of the drug also determines the frequency of administration.
- With regards to efficacy, administration via the subcutaneous route using short-acting ESAs required up to 30% less drug to be administered to achieve the same Hb/Hct.

RECOMMENDATIONS

R30   The patient with anaemia of CKD and the prescriber should agree (and revise as appropriate) the route of administration of ESAs, taking into account the following factors:
- patient population (eg haemodialysis patients)
- pain of injection
- frequency of administration
- the lifestyle and preferences of the patient
- efficacy (eg subcutaneous vs intravenous administration, or long-acting vs short-acting preparations)
- cost of drug supply.   (C)

R31   The prescriber should take into account that when using short-acting ESAs, subcutaneous injection allows the use of lower doses of drugs than intravenous administration.   (A)

6.8 ESAs: dose and frequency

6.8.1 Clinical introduction

Currently, the available ESAs fall into two broad classes, short- and long-acting. The characteristics of long-acting ESAs are such that when using these agents the shortest dose interval is weekly, with no appreciable difference between subcutaneous and intravenous routes of administration. With short-acting ESAs, dose intervals of a week or more are less cost effective than shorter dose intervals, and the subcutaneous route of administration is more cost effective than the intravenous route.

In patients without renal disease, studies looking at erythropoietin response to anaemia show an exponential rise in serum EPO levels with falling haemoglobin, suggesting that with increasing severity of anaemia the natural 'endogenous' EPO dose is initially high and subsequently tails off as the anaemia corrects. Although it would be logical to attempt to mimic this, the early days of ESA therapy showed that very rapid correction of anaemia was associated with significant adverse effects. The dose and frequency of administration of ESA is therefore likely to depend on haemoglobin level and rate of change of haemoglobin, the class of ESA used and (in the case of short-acting ESAs) the route of administration, the CKD population under treatment, and various patient factors and patient preferences.

6.8.2 Methodological introduction

A literature search identified nine studies.[188–196]

Two studies[197,198] had methodological limitations and were therefore excluded from the evidence statements. As the meta-analysis[198] addressing route of administration had methodological limitations, the 10 studies within it were individually appraised and five met quality criteria.[132,170,172,175,199]

The clinically relevant factors and respective study types are detailed in Table 6.3.

Table 6.3 Summary of included studies	
Route of administration	**Study design**
Studies included in the meta-analysis	
132	RCT
170	RCT
172	RCT
175	RCT
199	Cohort study
Study published after the meta-analysis literature search cut-off date	
188	Cohort study

continued

Table 6.3 Summary of included studies – *continued*

Starting Hb level	Study design
189	Prospective longitudinal study
Hypertension	**Study design**
190	Before and after study
191	RCT (open-label)
Rate of Hb correction	**Study design**
192	Prospective longitudinal study
193	Retrospective longitudinal study
194	Cohort study
195	Prospective longitudinal study
196	RCT(open-label)

The GDG agreed that the outcomes of priority were Hb levels, rate of Hb correction and complications.

Notable aspects of the evidence base were:

- Due to methodological limitations, one RCT[191] was downgraded to Level 2 in the evidence hierarchy.
- Adjuvant red blood cell transfusions were administered in addition to epoetin during the study period in four studies.[172,189,195,196]
- Two studies addressing rate of Hb correction[193,195] were conducted in children.

6.8.3 Evidence statements

▷ Route of administration

Table 6.4 Haemodialysis patients

Study reference	Evidence hierarchy	ESA therapy arms	Outcome
188	Level 2++	Once weekly s.c. vs once weekly i.v.	• The number of patients who maintained a stable Hb level (defined as a decrease of ≤1 g/dl) was similar in both groups. • Decrease ($p<0.05$) in Hb concentration in the i.v. treated group when the evaluation phase of the study was compared with the dosing phase. • Increased ($p<0.05$) mean weekly dose of epoetin alfa needed to maintain individual target Hb levels in the i.v. group.

continued

Table 6.4 Haemodialysis patients – *continued*

Study reference	Evidence hierarchy	ESA therapy arms	Outcome
172	Level 1++	Three times weekly i.v. vs three times weekly s.c.	• Hb and Hct were similar in both groups. • Average weekly epoetin dose was lower (p=0.002) in the s.c. group.
175	Level 1++	s.c. vs i.v.	• Mean Hb levels were stable and remained equivalent in both groups at the end of the study. • Epoetin requirement was found to be less (p=0.02) when administered by the s.c. route. When the different dosing strata were studied (ie >150 U/kg/week vs 100–150 U/kg/week vs <100 U/kg/week), it was evident that this difference was only in patients with the highest epoetin needs (>150 U/kg/wk).
199	Level 2+	s.c. vs i.v.	• Hct levels were similar over the entire study period.
170	Level 1+	Three times weekly s.c. vs three times weekly i.v.	• Weight-standardised epoetin doses at monthly intervals and cumulative epoetin doses were similar in both groups. • Hct levels were similar in both groups.
132	Level 1+	Three times weekly s.c. vs three times weekly i.v.	• Although time to reach the target Hb was longer (p=0.037) in the i.v. treated group, mean Hb and Hct levels were similar in both groups. • Epoetin requirement was greater (p=0.019) in the i.v. group during the Hb stabilisation phase of the study, but once target Hb was achieved in both groups, no difference was observed between the two groups.

A meta-analysis of the four Level 1 studies addressing epoetin dose when administered s.c. vs i.v.[132,170,172,175] found a lower epoetin requirement when administered s.c. (weighted mean difference (WMD) –30.05 (95% CI –43.96 to –16.14) I^2 =7%). This was in support of the findings of the excluded heterogeneous meta-analysis.[198] A sensitivity analysis excluding the study with sample size n <20[170] was also in agreement with this finding and ruled out heterogeneity (WMD –41.61 (95% CI –60.66 to –22.55) I^2 =0%).

Table 6.5 Starting Hb level

Study reference	Patient population	Evidence hierarchy	Hb level at baseline	Outcome
189	Continuous ambulatory peritoneal dialysis (CAPD)	Level 3	≤7.5 g/dl vs >7.5 g/dl	• Time to achieve Hb target was longer (p<0.001) in the lower Hb group at 6 months despite similar rate of Hb increase and epoetin dose in both groups.
195	Children on haemodialysis	Level 3 vs ≥6.8 g/dl	<6.8 g/dl	• A similar proportion of each group (81% vs 80%) reached the target Hb of 9.6–11.2 g/dl. • The median time to achieve target Hb was higher in the lower Hb group (median 13 weeks vs 9 weeks; p-value not reported by the authors).

Table 6.6 Hypertension: haemodialysis patients

Study reference	Evidence hierarchy	ESA therapy arms	Outcome
190	Level 3	i.v. three times weekly	• No change in mean systolic and diastolic blood pressures was found, and only three of 24 patients who had required treatment for hypertension before epoetin therapy required an increased dose of antihypertensive medication.
191	Level 2+	Hct 40.8 ± 5.2% vs Hct 30 ± 4.3%	• No differences were found in mean daytime systolic or diastolic BP and mean night time systolic or diastolic BP between the two groups.

Table 6.7 Rate of Hb correction

Study reference	Patient population	Evidence hierarchy	ESA therapy	Outcome
192	Predialysis	Level 3	s.c. twice weekly	• There was a rise in Hb and Hct when compared with baseline levels after 3 months, which was sustained after 6 months and 12 months (all p<0.001). • Target Hb was achieved 10–11 g/dl after 6 months.

continued

Table 6.7 Rate of Hb correction

Study reference	Patient population	Evidence hierarchy	ESA therapy	Outcome
195	Children on haemodialysis	Level 3	i.v. two to three times weekly with an aim to achieve a rise in Hb of 1 g/dl per 4 weeks in order to attain target Hb 9.6–11.2 g/dl	• A median time to target of 11 weeks was achieved with a median dose of 150 U/kg/week in 81% of patients. The mean rate of Hb rise was 0.5 g/dl per 4 weeks in patients receiving the starting dose of 75 U/kg/week and 0.8 g/dl per 4 weeks in those whose dose had been increased to 150 U/kg/week (p value not reported by the authors).
194	Haemodialysis	Level 2+	Same weekly epoetin alfa dose in varying dose intervals	• Patients who received 4,000 U epoetin as a bolus injection did not require increased epoetin doses, but dosing intervals significantly increased (p=0.01), unlike patients who received 10,000 U epoetin at intervals who required higher epoetin doses (p=0.002) with reduced dosing intervals (p=0.0001) to maintain Hb >11 g/dl throughout the 24-week study period.
196	Peritoneal dialysis patients	Level 1+	5, 10 and 20 U/kg epoetin daily s.c., to target Hct 30–35%	• The differences in the mean weekly change in Hct were significant (p<0.05) over the 8 week constant-dose phase, between all three groups, in ascending order. • During the correction phase, the time to achieve the target Hct in 50% of the patients (total n=72) who received 5, 10 and 20 U/kg daily s.c. was 154, 119 and 92 days respectively and the median cumulative epoetin doses to reach target Hct were calculated as 1,494, 1,523 and 1,678 U/kg respectively.
193	Post-transplant paediatric patients with chronic allograft dysfunction	Level 3	Thrice weekly s.c. vs twice weekly s.c. vs once weekly s.c.	• There was an increased Hct in 84% of the children from 23.2% ± 3.1% to 33% ± 3.1% (p value not reported by the authors) within 7.2 ± 4.9 weeks at a mean rate of 1.98% per week. • Hct increase and epoetin starting dose were linearly related (r=0.44, p<0.05).

6.8.4 Health economics methodological introduction

One study[200] was identified in a literature search. Three studies[149,198,201] did not meet quality criteria. The included study[200] estimated the increased costs of changing from s.c. epoetin to i.v. epoetin in a retrospective analysis of 99 haemodialysis patients over 7 months.

A cost-minimisation analysis was conducted at the request of the GDG to compare subcutaneous and intravenous epoetin administration. Full details are given in Appendix D.[*]

6.8.5 Evidence statements

The mean dose in the 's.c. switched to i.v.' patients increased significantly (46.83 + 10.20 IU/kg/week, +34.9%, p=0.001) over 7 months and was estimated to increase costs by €1,841 + €401 (Euros, 2002) per patient per year (+26.3%).[200]

The cost-minimisation analysis presented to the GDG stated in conclusion: 'The subcutaneous route of administration of epoetin vs intravenous route results in cost savings of approximately £1,100 + £727 per patient per year'.

6.8.6 From evidence to recommendations

Of the factors addressed, hypertension was not shown to have an effect in determining the dose and frequency of ESAs required to correct anaemia. But the route of administration and the rate of correction were important factors.

An acceptable rate of rise of haemoglobin was considered to be ~1–2g/dl/month. In general, it was thought that a patient's pre-treatment starting level of Hb would not influence the starting dose of ESA, but that their subsequent haemoglobin response would influence the dose thereafter.

Hypertension should be treated prior to the administration of ESAs. It was stated that episodes of severe hypertension would temporarily alter the dose of ESA, but that generally hypertension would not affect this issue.

The included health economic study supported the excluded meta-analysis[198] that intravenous administration of short-acting ESAs was more costly than subcutaneous administration.

The group concluded that in general s.c. administration leads to a reduced dose of short acting ESA. One study indicated that this was only relevant during the stabilisation phase but not during the maintenance phase of treatment.

RECOMMENDATION

R32   When correcting anaemia of CKD, the dose and frequency of ESAs should be:
- determined by the duration of action and route of administration of the ESA   (B)
- adjusted to keep the rate of Hb increase between 1 and 2g/dl/month.   (D(GPP))

---

[*] In interpreting economic evaluation of ESAs, it should be borne in mind that different units will have developed their own pricing structures which may differ considerably from BNF list prices.

6.9 Optimal Hb levels

6.9.1 Clinical introduction

The optimal haemoglobin range to be maintained following correction of anaemia associated with CKD is that which confers the most benefit and least adverse effect in the most cost-effective way.

The key questions are:

- Do patients with higher haemoglobin levels do well because they are less sick, and is it because they are less sick that they attain higher haemoglobin levels?
- Or is there a causal relationship between higher haemoglobin levels and lower risks of morbidity and mortality, and if so what is the optimal haemoglobin range to be maintained?

6.9.2 Clinical methodological introduction

A literature search identified one meta-analysis[202] containing 19 RCTs, which assessed the effects of lower vs higher haemoglobin collectively in predialysis, peritoneal dialysis and haemodialysis patients attained by means of ESA therapy or blood transfusion. The findings were stratified into two categories, namely studies that compared treatment to two haemoglobin ranges, higher (11.9–15.0 g/dl) vs lower (9.0–12.0 g/dl) (seven studies) and those which assessed the effects of epoetin (Hb 9.5–13.3 g/dl) vs no treatment (Hb 7.5–10.4 g/dl) (12 studies).

An additional three RCTs[203–205] and a prospective longitudinal study[206] were found which addressed the effects of lower vs higher Hb levels.

The different Hb levels examined and study durations need to be accounted for when evaluating the evidence and are summarised in Table 6.8.

Table 6.8 Study duration and Hb levels for the included studies			
Reference	Study duration	Low Hb (g/dl)	High Hb (g/dl)
202	6 to 29 months	9.0–12.0	11.9–15.0
202	2 to 12 months	7.5–10.4	9.5–13.3
204	8 months	9.0	12.0
205	24 months	10.9 ± 0.7	12.6 ± 1.0
206	8 months	10.5 ± 0.9	13.4 ± 3.1

Notable aspects of the evidence base were:

- Although the meta-analysis[202] was of rigorous methodology leading to a systematic review of a high standard, the trials within it were of variable quality.
- The meta-analysis[202] was heavily weighted by a single study[207] conducted in haemodialysis patients with severe cardiovascular disease, which may imply unsuitability for extrapolation to the entire CKD patient population.

- Although two studies in the meta-analysis[202] enrolled children, the findings were not stratified on the basis of age.
- Due to methodology limitations, one RCT[204] was downgraded to Level 2+ of the evidence hierarchy.
- The means of achieving target Hb in the studies included the use of ESAs and/or blood transfusions.

6.9.3   Clinical evidence statements

Table 6.9 Summary of appraised studies

Reference	Outcome	Patient population (n)	Aiming for a high Hb	Aiming for a low Hb	Evidence grading
202	All-cause mortality	Predialysis, peritoneal dialysis and haemodialysis (n=1949)	11.9–15.0g/dl	9.0–12.0 g/dl ↓	Level 1++
202	All-cause mortality	Predialysis, peritoneal dialysis and haemodialysis (n=255)	9.5–13.3 g/dl	7.5–10.4 g/dl No difference	Level 1++
202	Hypertension	Predialysis, peritoneal dialysis and haemodialysis (n=1277)	11.9–15.0 g/dl	9.0–12.0 g/dl No difference	Level 1++
203	Hypertension	Haemodialysis (n=12)	12.0 g/dl ↑	9.0 g/dl	Level 2+
202	Quality of life	Predialysis, peritoneal dialysis and haemodialysis (n=unknown)	11.9–15.0 g/dl	9.0–12.0 g/dl No difference	Level 1++
202	Quality of life	Predialysis, peritoneal dialysis and haemodialysis (n=unknown)	9.5–13.3 g/dl	7.5–10.4 g/dl No difference	Level 1++
204	Quality of life	Haemodialysis (n=12)	12.0 g/dl	9.0 g/dl No difference	Level 2+
203	Physical performance-exercise radionuclide ventriculogram	Haemodialysis (n=12)	12.0 g/dl	9.0 g/dl No difference	Level 2+
203	Physical performance-maximal incremental exercise testing	Haemodialysis (n=12)	12.0 g/dl ↑	9.0 g/dl	Level 2+
205	6-minute walking distance	Haemodialysis (n=596)	12.6 ± 1.0 g/dl	10.9 ± 0.7 g/dl No difference	Level 1++
203	Left ventricular mass and mass index	Haemodialysis (n=12)	12.0 g/dl	9.0 g/dl No difference (note: short study duration)	Level 2+

continued

Table 6.9 Summary of appraised studies – *continued*

Reference	Outcome	Patient population (n)	Aiming for a high Hb	Aiming for a low Hb	Evidence grading
205	Left ventricular volume index, left ventricular mass index	Haemodialysis (n=596)	12.6 ± 1.0 g/dl	10.9 ± 0.7 No difference in either cardiovascular parameter	Level 1++
206	Left ventricular septal, posterior wall thickness and left ventricular mass index Left ventricular ESD and EDD RWT parameter for left ventricular geometry	Haemodialysis patients with LVH and enhanced LVMI at baseline (n=23)	13.4 ± 3.1 g/dl All ↓ No difference ↓	10.5 ± 0.9 g/dl	Level 3

↑ = significant increase; ↓ = significant decrease.

6.9.4 Health economics methodological introduction

A cost-utility analysis study was appraised, which estimated the incremental cost per QALY of treating haemodialysis patients with epoetin doses adjusted to attain haemoglobin target ranges of 9.5 to 10.5 g/dl, 11.0 to 12.0 g/dl, 12.0 to 12.5 g/dl and 14.0 g/dl.[208]

An economic model was constructed to evaluate the cost effectiveness of various haemoglobin ranges in haemodialysis patients. Full details are given in Appendix C.[*]

6.9.5 Health economics evidence statements

An additional $55,295 per additional QALY gained (95% CI: $51,404–$59,822) was required to achieve the target haemoglobin range of 11.0–12.0 g/dl vs a 9.5–10.5 g/dl haemoglobin target range.[208]

An additional $613,015 per additional QALY gained (95% CI: $569,884–$663,210) was required to achieve the target haemoglobin range of 12.0–12.5 g/dl vs a 11.0–12.0 g/dl haemoglobin target range.[208]

An additional $828,215 per additional QALY gained (95% CI: $769,942–$896,030) was required to achieve the target haemoglobin of 14.0 g/dl vs a 12.0–12.5 g/dl haemoglobin target range.[208]

The dose of epoetin and the estimate of health-related quality of life had the largest effect on results in the sensitivity analysis, assuming 32% (base-case assumes 14%) lower dose requirement for subcutaneous epoetin than intravenous epoetin:

---

[*] In interpreting economic evaluation of ESAs, it should be borne in mind that different units will have developed their own pricing structures which may differ considerably from BNF list prices.

Table 6.10 Target Hb levels and incremental cost per QALY

Target Hb	Incremental cost per QALY
11.0–12.0 g/dl vs 9.5–10.5 g/dl	$38,340
12.0–12.5 g/dl vs 11.0–12.0 g/dl	$423,174
14.0 g/dl vs 12.0–12.5 g/dl	$569,500

▷ Health economic modelling

The economic model presented to the GDG stated in conclusion: 'The results suggest that treating anaemia with a target Hb 11–12 g/dl is cost effective in haemodialysis patients based on a £30,000 (incremental cost-effectiveness ratio) threshold. However, there is uncertainty in the results of the model from lack of certainty in the input parameters. Nevertheless, the results are relatively robust based on one-way sensitivity analyses and threshold analyses. This analysis is a simplified model of the costs and benefits of treating anaemia in the haemodialysis population and a variety of assumptions have been used in the baseline analysis'. See Appendix C for details.

6.9.6 From evidence to recommendations

The GDG noted that the largest meta-analysis considered was heavily skewed by one study that influenced the data on mortality.[202] This study of patients with cardiovascular disease was terminated early because of a trend towards increased mortality in the high target haemoglobin group. Thus statistical significance between the two groups could not be achieved. The GDG accepted that most of the studies it contained did not state their method of randomisation and were not adequately blinded; only two were carried out on an intention to treat basis.[202] It was noted that a target Hb level of 14 ± 1 g/dl (converted from Hct) was associated with higher mortality in a study of patients with congestive heart failure and ischaemic heart disease. The GDG thought this may have related to the large doses of iron and epoetin that had to be administered in order for a sicker patient to achieve a haemoglobin in this range.[202] It was considered unhelpful both clinically and economically to administer increasing doses of epoetin and iron to a patient who was not responding adequately to the treatment. The GDG agreed with the authors of the meta-analysis that it would be prudent to ensure that patients with cardiovascular impairment maintain a Hb below 12.0 g/dl.

The GDG did not feel that increasing age should be a specific factor in setting a haemoglobin target but felt that low levels of physical activity in some individuals should be considered before setting the haemoglobin range for that individual.

The GDG highlighted that two studies within the meta-analysis[202] included children but that no outcome data were specifically reported from this population. The GDG noted that despite a lack of direct evidence relating to children, they could in general be expected to benefit from a similar Hb level to adults.

The GDG noted that the kinetics of a patient's response to epoetin vary. This means that whatever range of haemoglobin is specified as being optimal, it is inevitable that some patients will have a haemoglobin outside this range some of the time. This is because action to maintain the haemoglobin within the specified range may only be taken when a haemoglobin measurement falls outside the range and it will take time for any action to produce an effect. The GDG therefore agreed that they would specify a target range in the knowledge that this would result in most patients maintaining a haemoglobin concentration within 0.5g/dl either side of that specified range.

The GDG felt that setting a Hb range of 11.0–12.0g/dl would in effect allow the majority of patients to reach a level between 10.5 and 12.5 g/dl. It was noted from anecdotal evidence that maintaining a Hb of 12g/dl could make a large difference to a patients quality of life, exercise capacity and cognitive function; the increase in physical performance was further supported by the evidence.[203] The GDG also considered a health economic model that suggested haemoglobin ranges above 12 g/dl were not cost effective because of the high cost of epoetin and low incremental QALYs gained from higher haemoglobin ranges.[208]

The consensus among the GDG was that a range of 11.0–12.0 g/dl was consistent with both the clinical and health economic evidence.

RECOMMENDATIONS

R33   In people with anaemia of CKD, treatment should maintain stable haemoglobin (Hb) levels between 10.5 and 12.5 g/dl for adults and children older than 2 years of age, and between 10 and 12 g/dl in children younger than 2 years of age, reflecting the lower normal range in that age group. This should be achieved by:

- Adjusting treatment, typically when Hb rises above 12.0 or falls below 11.0 g/dl.
- Taking patient preferences, symptoms and comorbidities into account and revising the aspirational range and action thresholds accordingly.   (C)

R34   In people who do not achieve a haemoglobin level above 10.5g/dl (or 10.0 g/dl in children younger than 2 years of age) despite correction of iron deficiency and exclusion of the known causes of resistance to ESA therapy (defined as treatment with ≥300 IU/kg/week of subcutaneous epoetin or ≥450IU/kg/week of intravenous epoetin or 1.5µg/kg/week of darbepoetin), lower levels of haemoglobin may have to be accepted.   (D(GPP))

R35   Age alone should not be a determinant for treatment of anaemia of CKD.   (D(GPP))

See 3.2.3 for the associated algorithm.

6.10 Optimum haemoglobin levels in children with anaemia of CKD

6.10.1 Methodological introduction

The two RCTs reported in the meta-analysis[202] conducted in children[209,210] – one of cross-over design[210] – were used to address the effects of lower vs higher haemoglobin and were individually appraised. An additional cross-over RCT[211] that was conducted in the same paediatric population was also appraised.

Issues for consideration were as follows:

- The two cross-over RCTs[211,210] were downgraded to Level 2+ because of methodological limitations.
- One study[209] had set out to investigate dosing requirements.
- Study duration to assess cardiovascular benefits of epoetin administration[211] may not have been sufficiently long at 48 weeks.

Table 6.11 Summary characteristics of appraised studies

Study	N	Target Hb	Study type	Study duration
209	44	Between mean and 2 standard deviations below mean for age	RCT of low dose vs high dose epoetin	12 weeks
211	7	10.5–12.0 g/dl	Cross-over RCT of epoetin vs placebo	24 weeks in each limb, 48 weeks total
210	7	10.5–12.0 g/dl	Cross-over RCT of epoetin vs placebo	24 weeks in each limb, 48 weeks total

6.10.2 Evidence statements

Table 6.12 Evidence statements for optimum Hb levels in children

Study	Hypertension and cardiovascular parameters	Patient population (n)	Achieved high Hb	Achieved low Hb	Evidence grading
209	Systolic and diastolic BP No difference	Children on haemodialysis, peritoneal dialysis and predialysis (n=44)	12.9 ± 0.7; 11.9 ± 1.6; 12.7 ± 2.0 g/dl	8.4 ± 1.0; 10 ± 2.04; 11.9 ± 1.8 g/dl	Level 1+
211	Cardiac index (p=0.01), ventricular stroke index (p=0.03),heart rate (p=0.002), aortic stroke distance (p=0.01), minute distance (p=0.03) and left ventricular end diastolic diameter (p=0.04) all decreased. There was no change in shortening fraction, interventricular septum and left ventricular posterior wall thickness. No change was found in systolic, diastolic or mean BP.	Children on peritoneal dialysis (n=7)	11.5 g/dl (target 10.5–12.0 g/dl)	6.9 g/dl	Level 2+

continued

Table 6.12 Evidence statements for optimum Hb levels in children – *continued*

Study	Exercise testing and quality of life	Patient population (n)	Achieved high Hb	Achieved low Hb	Evidence grading
210	No changes were found in the 2-minute walking distance (n=7) and treadmill exercise testing workload (n=3). A reduction in heart rate at rest was found after epoetin administration (p=0.02) and at each successive stage of the exercise test. No arrhythmias or ischaemic changes were found.	Children on peritoneal dialysis (n=7)	Median 11.2 g/dl (range 9.5–14.2 g/dl)	Median 7.3 g/l (range 4.2–8.1 g/l)	Level 2+
210	Quality of life (25-part parental questionnaire, using a visual analogue scale) found an improvement in physical performance and general health (p<0.02), but the global score did not find an improvement in quality of life.	Children on peritoneal dialysis (n=7)	Median 11.2 g/dl (range 9.5–14.2 g/dl)	Median 7.3 g/l (range 4.2–8.1 g/l)	Level 2+

6.10.3 From evidence to recommendations

The use of exercise testing for outcomes is not meaningful in very young children, which exacerbates the problem of the small sample size in the evidence.

RECOMMENDATIONS

Recommendations pertaining to children with anaemia of chronic kidney disease are presented in relevant sections throughout the guideline.

6.11 Adjusting ESA therapy

6.11.1 Clinical introduction

ESA dose adjustments are made to encourage haemoglobin levels into the recommended ranges. The details of such 'targeting' varies unit by unit, but must always involve decisions on when to make the dose change (ie at what haemoglobin level), and by how much to change the ESA dose and/or frequency. ESA therapy (even with the currently available long-acting agent) involves delivery of short, intermittent, pharmacological bursts of bioavailable EPO which bear no relation, either temporally or in magnitude, to normal physiological control of erythropoiesis. Under normal conditions, the body's oxygen sensing, EPO-producing, and erythropoietic systems are closely regulated and coordinated to maintain haemoglobin levels within a narrow range. During ESA therapy, haemoglobin levels fluctuate widely and the pattern of fluctuation varies from patient to patient.[212] This haemoglobin cycling may complicate the management of anaemia associated with CKD. Factors likely to be associated with fluctuations in haemoglobin level include changes in ESA dose, intravenous iron treatment, intercurrent illness (especially infection) and hospitalisation. Those patients experiencing more frequent fluctuations, and those with the greatest amplitude of fluctuation, have been characterised as being more responsive to ESAs.[213]

Experimental and clinical studies have defined a desirable outcome range of haemoglobin and have used the limits of the range to trigger a dose change when the haemoglobin level falls above or below these limits. The extent of the dose change, whether an absolute amount or a proportion of the existing dose, has to fit the available ESA formulations or decisions are required about the dosage interval. However, because of logistical delays in responding to any current laboratory value and because of differences in the momentum of haemoglobin change, it may be necessary to alter ESA therapy pre-emptively prior to the haemoglobin level breaching the limits of the desirable range. There are also individual variations in the response to ESAs that may be taken into account from historical data. The case mix and treatment history of any patient cohort will also influence the outcome and while tailoring of the timing and dose changes may be attempted there is inevitable unpredictability of outcome.

So how then do we adjust ESA dose and dose frequency to keep haemoglobin levels within the maintenance range, and what factors determine how we do this?

6.11.2 Clinical methodological introduction

A literature search found 13 studies: an RCT,[214] prospective cohort studies,[215,216] retrospective cohort studies,[217–219] cross-over studies,[220,221] retrospective longitudinal studies,[222,223] and cross-sectional studies.[224–226]

One study[187] had methodological limitations and was therefore excluded from the evidence statements.

6.11.3 Clinical evidence statements

▷   Factors affecting epoetin dose: route of epoetin administration

Haemodialysis patients

One study[222] found patients administered with epoetin by the i.v. route received significantly higher doses than those prescribed epoetin by the s.c. route (p=0.0001). (**Level 3**)

▷   Iron status

Haemodialysis patients

Three studies found epoetin dose to be inversely correlated with iron status when measured by means of serum transferrin saturation (p=0.0001),[222] serum saturation ratio (r=-0.16, p=0.003)[224] and total iron binding capacity levels (r=0.27, p<0.01).[219] (**Level 3 and Level 2+**)

In contrast, one study[219] did not find an association with serum transferrin saturation. Also, no association between epoetin dose and serum ferritin levels was found in two studies.[219,222] (**Level 3 and Level 2+**)

▷ Dialysis adequacy

Haemodialysis patients

One study[222] found an inverse correlation between urea reduction ratio and administered epoetin dose (p<0.0001). (**Level 3**)

▷ Cause of end stage renal failure

Haemodialysis patients

One study[222] found diabetes mellitus as the cause of end stage renal failure to be associated with lower epoetin doses (p=0.003). (**Level 3**)

▷ Inflammation

Haemodialysis patients

One study[224] found a direct correlation between administered epoetin dose and malnutrition-inflammation score (ie increasing degree of severity) (r=0.13, p=0.03). This was reflected in the direct correlation between weekly epoetin dose and logarithmic inflammatory cytokines, IL-6 (r=0.31, p<0.001) and TNF-α (r=0.18, 0.001) as well as C-reactive protein (CRP) (r=0.18, p<0.001) and lactase (p<0.001) levels. Similarly, there was an inverse correlation observed between epoetin dose and nutritional markers (r=-0.19, p<0.001).

In another study,[225] albumin (r=-0.359, p<0.001), log CRP (r=0.337, p=0.001), log ferritin (r=0.240, p=0.021) and transferrin (r=−0.264, p=0.011) all showed correlation with epoetin:Hct ratio. When patients in the lowest and highest epoetin:Hct quartiles were compared, only median CRP showed statistical significance (p=0.009). (**Level 3**)

Contrary to the above findings, in one study[226] C-reactive protein levels did not show any association with epoetin dose. (**Level 3**)

Peritoneal dialysis patients

In one study,[225] albumin (r=-0.453, p=0.006) and CRP (r=0.375, p=0.024) showed correlation with epoetin/Hct ratio, but not ferritin. (**Level 3**)

Haemodialysis vs peritoneal dialysis patients

When compared with one another in the same study,[225] haemodialysis patients had a greater epoetin/Hct ratio than peritoneal dialysis patients (p<0.001), which was matched with a higher epoetin dose (p<0.001) and lower Hct levels (p=0.002). Also lower CRP (p<0.001), ferritin (p<0.001), transferrin (p<0.001) and aluminium (p<0.001) levels were found in the haemodialysis patients. However, no difference was observed for albumin, transferrin saturation, intact parathyroid hormone and PCRn. (**Level 3**)

▷ Adjunctive medical treatment

Haemodialysis patients

Higher epoetin doses were administered to patients receiving ACE-inhibitor therapy when compared with those not treated with ACE-inhibitors (p<0.05) in one study.[219] In a 12-month study,[216] patients receiving high dose enalapril (ACE-inhibitor) required a higher epoetin dose at the end of the study period (p<0.0001) and also when compared with those receiving nifedipine (calcium-channel blocker) (p<0.0001) or control (epoetin only) (p<0.0001) to maintain a Hb >10 g/dl. Similarly, in a 12-month study aimed to maintain Hb >10 g/dl,[215] high dose losartan (angiotensin-II receptor blocker) required a higher epoetin dose at the end of the study period (p<0.0001) and also when compared with those receiving amlodipine (calcium-channel blocker) (p<0.0001) or control (epoetin only) (p<0.0001). (**Level 2+**)

In contrast to the above findings, two studies with patients receiving ACE-inhibitors[217,220] aimed to maintain Hct levels at 30–36% (Hb ~ 10–12 g/dl) did not find any association between ACE-inhibitor administration and epoetin resistance. (**Level 2+**)

Peritoneal dialysis patients

Weekly epoetin dose given to maintain Hct >30% (Hb ~ 10 g/dl) at the end of a 12-week study[214] was greater in patients receiving ACE-inhibitors (p<0.01) and in patients receiving angiotensin-II receptor blocker treatment (p<0.05), but not in those receiving calcium-channel blockers when compared with individual weekly doses at the beginning of the study. In addition, plasma epoetin levels were higher in the ACE-inhibitor treated group (p<0.05) but not in the angiotensin-II receptor blocker and control groups. (**Level 1+**)

▷ Parathyroid hormone

Haemodialysis patients

In a study conducted in patients over the age of 65 years, whereby patients were divided into PTH >250 pg/ml and <250 pg/ml, despite similar epoetin doses and serum iron and ferritin levels, patients in the hyperparathyroid group had lower Hb and Hct levels (p=0.009 and p=0.008 respectively) as well as higher levels of alkaline phosphatase (p=0.023), phosphorus (p=0.001) and calcium x phosphorus product (p=0.009).[221] (**Level 2+**)

▷ Hospitalisation

Haemodialysis patients

In one study,[223] higher epoetin doses were required in patients who were transfused during hospitalisation up to 2 months following discharge (p<0.05). (**Level 3**)

The same study[223] found no association between discharge diagnosis, (inflammatory vs non-inflammatory) or surgical procedure during hospitalisation and epoetin requirement up to 2 months following discharge. (**Level 3**)

▷ Dialysate chloramine levels

Haemodialysis patients

One before and after study (n=72)[227] found an association between higher achieved Hb level (p<0.001) and decreased epoetin dose (p<0.001) with installation of new carbon filters, which decreased the chloramine levels from to 0.25 parts per million (ppm) to <0.1 ppm. This was supported by findings in a subgroup analysis (n=15) that showed low-grade haemolysis by a post-dialysis rise in methaemoglobins (p<0.01) and a drop in haptoglobins (p<0.01), which was not detected after the use of the carbon filters. Additionally, the water board confirmed the sustained two fold increase in chloramines levels and acceptable levels of nitrate, aluminium, bacterial counts and endotoxins in the mains water supply during the study time period. In agreement, one satellite dialysis unit,[218] found decreasing Hb levels at months 10 (p<0.01) and 11 (p<0.01) of the study despite higher epoetin dose (p=0.04) when compared with other local dialysis units. These findings were associated with a high chlorine water content relative to the desirable limit (p value not given), which coincided with evidence of haemolysis as shown by higher ferritin (p<0.01) and low haptoglobin (p value not given). Furthermore, installation of an activated charcoal filter decreased chlorine concentration to <0.02, which was accompanied by an increase in Hb and a reduction in epoetin requirement. (**Level 2+ and Level 3**)

6.11.4 Health economics methodological introduction

The appraised study[228] performed a decision analysis comparing three dosage regimens: epoetin-6 strategy, 6,000 U (107 U/kg), epoetin-9 strategy, 9,000 U (167 U/kg) and epoetin-12 strategy, 12,000 U (211 U/kg) of subcutaneous epoetin in continuous ambulatory peritoneal dialysis to maintain the target Hct level of 0.33 (equivalent to 11 g/dl).[228] Epoetin was given weekly for the first 2 months until a target Hct of 0.33 was reached. This was maintained for an additional 3 months with the administration frequency reduced to fortnightly or 4-weekly. Non-responders in 6,000 U and 9,000 U after 2 months entered 12,000 U regimen.

6.11.5 Health economics evidence statements

Of the three subcutaneous epoetin strategies compared, it was most cost effective in peritoneal dialysis patients to give 6,000 units weekly for 2 months, followed by a weekly or 2-weekly epoetin 6,000 unit dose for the next 3 months while maintaining the target Hct level of 0.33 and to restart non-responders after 2 months on the 12,000 unit epoetin strategy.[228] The savings from the lower administration frequency of the 9,000 unit dosage regime were offset by the higher cumulative acquisition cost.[228]

Varying the parameters over the 20-week treatment period:
- Epoetin-6 strategy is always the least costly over the $0–60 range for drug administration costs. Drug administration costs must be $137 for epoetin-6 to become more costly than epoetin-12.
- Epoetin-6 is least costly over the 95% CI range for response probabilities.
- Epoetin-12 strategy becomes less costly than the Epoetin-9 as drug administration costs increase over $35.

Varying the parameters over a 1-year treatment period:

- Epoetin-6 was less costly than both epoetin-9 and epoetin-12 over the range of costs ($0–60).
- Epoetin-6 becomes more costly than epoetin-12 at $95.
- Epoetin-6 was less costly over whole range of 95% CI.
- Epoetin-9 was more costly than epoetin-12 at lower 95%CI limit.
- Epoetin-12 becomes less costly than epoetin-9 at drug administration costs of $8 per injection and above.

6.11.6 From evidence to recommendations

Of all of the outcomes considered in the evidence, the GDG felt that the route of ESA administration, the patient's iron status, administration of adjunctive medical treatment, and the presence or absence of inflammation were of most relevance to determine the dose and frequency of ESA required to keep haemoglobin levels within the maintenance range in all CKD patients. Dose adjustments were also likely to be influenced by:

- the patient's haemoglobin level
- the observed rate of change in haemoglobin level
- an individual patient's response to ESA therapy.

In patients on haemodialysis, chloramine levels in dialysis water were also of relevance. The outcomes of dialysis adequacy, adjunctive medical treatment, race, and parathyroid hormone levels were discussed but the evidence was either limited or would be more fully covered in separate guideline sections, the GDG therefore did not wish to make any recommendations regarding these. The outcomes of end-stage renal failure and hospitalisation were included but the GDG did not feel that they were helpful in determining the dose and frequency of ESA required to keep haemoglobin levels within the maintenance range for individual patients.

With regards to the route of administration, two studies reported that doses of short-acting ESAs could be reduced when administered subcutaneously as opposed to intravenously.[187,222] It was noted that the decision of whether to administer ESAs s.c. or i.v. was also a matter of patient choice.

Several studies supported the view that the amount of ESA required is inversely correlated with iron status.[187,222,224] The GDG felt this was an important factor to take into account when determining the dose and frequency of ESA required to keep haemoglobin levels within the maintenance range and also Unit policy in view of the need for uniform and convenient clinical procedures.

The GDG noted that there was evidence to support a correlation between the weekly dose administration of ESA and inflammatory cytokines (IL-6, TNF-alfa).[224]

The GDG noted that the evidence supported the intuitive notion that sicker patients generally require higher doses of ESAs.[225] The GDG discussed that intercurrent illness may be a cause of temporary resistance that should be assessed, and it was noted that in patients with a chronic illness, resistance to ESAs may be prolonged.

The GDG discussed the evidence with respect to adjunctive medical treatment, that patients receiving either ACE inhibitor therapy or angiotensin-II receptor antagonists required an increased dose of ESA in comparison with those patients administered a calcium-channel blocker or to control groups.[215,219] Two further studies reported no association between ACE-inhibitor administration and resistance to ESAs.[217,220] The GDG considered one study to have methodological limitations due to the non-randomised study design.[220] The GDG noted that the treatment ranges in these studies were appropriate and the doses being administered would not lead the GDG to consider that ESA resistance should be suspected. The GDG concluded that there was no evidence that ACE-inhibitors caused ESA resistance and that such treatment should not be stopped, although the dose of ESA may require adjustment.

The GDG discussed the implications of dialysis water purity on ESA administration, in particular the GDG noted that increased chloramine levels (formed by the combination of free chlorine and ammonia gas) were associated with a need for higher doses of ESAs in haemodialysis patients.[218,227] The GDG discussed that the addition of activated charcoal filters reduced the level of chlorine in the dialysis water. However, it was noted that these filters can be prone to infection suggesting that a risk–benefit analysis would be useful. It was noted that neither study had performed such an analysis. The GDG noted that NHS Estates have produced a document covering facilities for renal services. This outlines that the required standards for water purity must be monitored and achieved (point 2.19), and specifically notes that 'carbon filters should be selected to achieve sufficient contact time to remove all chlorine and chloramines' (point 6.78).[229] This issue was considered an issue for a dialysis unit rather than the individual patient but the information may be of use to unit managers. The GDG concluded that dialysis units should consider the use of carbon filters but that a risk–benefit analysis should be used to assess the benefits of reducing chloramines levels against the risk of infection of the carbon filters.

The GDG discussed monitoring issues around how frequently patients should be monitored and when to intervene to correct the Hb level. It was felt that there was a need to follow the trend of a patient's response to Hb but that in general, if two consecutive tests taken a month apart fell outside the target range, or if the rate of rise or fall of haemoglobin exceeded 1 g/dl/month, then intervention would be necessary to correct the Hb level.

With regards to the health economic evidence, the GDG felt that there were some issues with the transferability of the costs from a study conducted in the USA to the UK healthcare setting. However, the GDG did agree with the principal message that giving a low dose of ESA more frequently was more cost effective at the unit level.

RECOMMENDATIONS

R36   Iron status should be optimised before or coincident with the initiation of ESA
        administration.   (C)

R37   Use of angiotensin-converting enzyme (ACE) inhibitors or angiotensin-II receptor
        antagonists is not precluded, but if they are used, an increase in ESA therapy should be
        considered.   (D)

R38   Haemoglobin measurements should be taken into account when determining the dose and frequency of ESA administration:

- The cause of an unexpected change in Hb level should be investigated (ie intercurrent illness, bleeding) to enable intervention.
- ESA dose and/or frequency should be increased or decreased when Hb measurements fall outside action thresholds (usually below 11.0g/dl or above 12.0g/dl), or for example when the rate of change of haemoglobin suggests an established trend (eg >1g/dl/month). (D(GPP))

See 3.2.3 for the associated algorithm.

6.12 Treating iron deficiency: correction

6.12.1 Clinical introduction

While there are many different preparations of oral iron available (see Table 6.13), there are currently only two forms of parenteral iron licensed in the UK, iron sucrose and iron dextran. The key issues are iron safety and efficacy.

Table 6.13 Iron content of different oral iron preparations		
Iron salt	Dose	Content of ferrous iron
Ferrous fumarate	200 mg	65 mg
Ferrous gluconate	300 mg	35 mg
Ferrous succinate	100 mg	35 mg
Ferrous sulphate	300 mg	60 mg
Ferrous sulphate, dried	200 mg	65 mg

Oral iron preparations contain varying amounts of ferrous iron, and the frequency of gastrointestinal side effects related to each different preparation tends to be directly related to the content of ferrous iron. Common adverse effects from oral preparations include constipation, diarrhoea, nausea, vomiting, and dyspepsia.

Iron sucrose is a complex of ferric hydroxide with sucrose containing 2% (20 mg/ml) of iron and iron dextran is a complex of ferric hydroxide with dextran containing 5% (50 mg/ml) of iron. Adverse effects from intravenous iron are mainly related to the size of dose and rate of infusion. Potential adverse effects include nausea, vomiting, abdominal pain, flushing, anaphylactoid reactions, dyspnoea, numbness, fever, urticaria, rash, arthralgia, myalgia, blurred vision, injection-site reactions including phlebitis, rarely diarrhoea, arrhythmias, hypotension, chest pain, seizures, tremor, dizziness, fatigue and sweating.

Intestinal iron absorption declines as serum ferritin increases[230,231] and ESA administration boosts iron absorption in erythropoietin deficient haemodialysis patients.[232] Patients with CKD who have anaemia, a GFR below 40 ml/min, and are not receiving ESA therapy are likely to be erythropoietin deficient.[72] The relative lack of oral iron efficacy in each of these conditions may be due to a lack of erythropoietin-stimulated iron absorption. This lack of oral iron efficacy led to the use of i.v. iron and early use of i.v. iron employed low doses given relatively frequently and administered as an infusion. Frequent administration of i.v. iron in haemodialysis patients is made feasible through use of dialysis vascular access but in peritoneal dialysis and predialysis patients venous access is required for each dose. Administration of higher doses in CKD patients not on haemodialysis offers the potential to spare venous access, but at the possible expense of increased adverse effects.

Relative to other CKD patient groups there is a wealth of information concerning iron status and response to iron administration in patients on haemodialysis. In CKD patients not on dialysis low iron indices are common. TSAT levels below 20% and ferritin levels below 100 µg/l may occur in up to 20–70% of patients, depending on CKD stage and gender [233] However, little is known about the relationship between baseline iron status, the likelihood of a response to an iron challenge, and the relative efficacy and safety of oral vs intravenous iron.

Iron therapy in haemodialysis patients is an essential adjuvant to ESA therapy and adequate iron stores are required prior to treatment with ESAs to ensure effective erythropoiesis. Virtually all haemodialysis patients will require ESA therapy to achieve target haemoglobin levels. By contrast, a significant proportion of predialysis CKD patients, and some peritoneal dialysis patients, may not require ESA therapy to achieve target haemoglobin levels. Iron therapy in these patients may be undertaken as primary treatment of anaemia.

6.12.2 Methodological introduction

A comprehensive literature search identified one RCT[234] investigating the efficacy of oral vs i.v. iron in predialysis patients without concurrent ESA therapy and two before and after studies investigating the efficacy of i.v. iron over 6 months[235] or as a single dose[236] in iron-deficient predialysis patients who had not previously received ESA therapy. A further before and after study was identified investigating the efficacy of i.v. iron over 12 months.[237]

One study[238] did not meet quality criteria and was therefore excluded from the evidence statements.

6.12.3 Evidence statements

▷ Iron dextran: predialysis patients

Following administration of 1g iron dextran in 500 ml normal saline i.v. as a total dose infusion over 6 hours (n=56), Hb (p<0.001) and serum ferritin (p<0.0001) levels increased after 12 weeks. However, this increase in Hb was not apparent after one year (n=21); ferritin was still increased compared with baseline, although to a lesser extent than at 12 weeks (p<0.001). In addition, no major adverse events were found and systolic and diastolic blood pressure did not change after 12 weeks.[236] (**Level 3**)

▷ Ferric saccharate (also known as ferric hydroxide sucrose or iron sucrose): predialysis patients

In one study 200 mg elemental iron (Ferric saccharate) was administered in 150 ml saline over 2 hours, once monthly for 5 months, to give a total i.v. iron dose of 1,000 mg per patient (n=33). After 3 months of i.v. iron treatment, the mean Hct and Hb values were not significantly increased, despite raised serum ferritin levels compared with baseline (p<0.05). At 6 months, however (ie 1 month after the last iron dose), the mean Hct (p=0.035) and Hb (p=0.008) had significantly increased. Additionally, there were no differences in those responding to i.v. iron treatment with an increase in mean Hct and Hb compared with those not responding in any of the other parameters (serum creatinine, creatinine clearance, systolic and diastolic blood pressure) either before or after onset of i.v. iron therapy. None of the patients reported side effects during the study period. Also, no correlation was found between Hb/Hct and any other of the study parameters in the responders and non-responders.[235] (**Level 3**)

In a study of pre-dialysed chronic renal failure patients with haemoglobin levels less than 11g/dl who were not receiving erythropoietin (n=60),[237] monthly intravenous administration of 200mg of iron sucrose for a period of 12 months was associated with a significant increase in haemoglobin from 9.7 ± 1.1 at baseline to 11.3 ± 2.5g/dl after 12 months (p<0.05): a mean increase of 1.6g/dl. No worsening of renal function, no increase in blood pressure and no other side effects were noted. (**Level 3**)

▷ Oral vs i.v. iron sucrose: predialysis patients

In a RCT[234] investigating i.v. iron sucrose 1,000mg in divided doses over 14 days administered either as an injection or infusion vs oral ferrous sulphate 325 mg three times daily (≡ 195 mg ferrous iron per day) for 56 days, in patients with and without ESA use, mean adherence of 97.3 (95% CI 94.3–100.0) in the i.v. treatment group was greater than in the oral treatment group mean 88.5 (95% CI 84.8–92.3). In addition, both the proportion of patients who achieved the primary end point (ie rise in Hb ≥1.0 g/dl) (p=0.0344) and the mean increase in Hb were higher in the i.v. group by day 42 (p=0.0298). Notably, the difference in ESA use in achieving primary end point in the i.v. and oral group was not found to be significant. Three patients in the i.v. group discontinued treatment due to adverse events attributed to the study drug (hypotension, n=2 and nausea, n=1). Transient taste disturbance (dysgeusia) was the most prominent GI complaint associated with i.v. iron administration. Constipation, diarrhoea, nausea, vomiting and dyspepsia were associated prominently with oral iron therapy, while headache, myalgia and hypotension were exclusively associated with i.v. iron administration. (**Level 1++**)

6.12.4 Health economics methodological introduction

One study was found but did not meet quality criteria.[239] The patient population contained three patients receiving epoetin, methodology of analysis was not stated, cost analysis was insufficiently reported and there was no estimation of uncertainty.

6.12.5 From evidence to recommendations

The available published evidence does not suggest the most effective and safest dose, frequency, preparation or route of administration of iron in ACKD patients with functional iron deficiency prior to ESA therapy. GDG consensus was that patients with anaemia associated with

CKD and functional iron deficiency will require intravenous iron treatment. The published evidence did not allow the GDG to recommend a preparation. Two preparations are available in the UK and the dose and frequency will be dictated by the preparation used and by measurement and monitoring of iron indices (serum ferritin and %HRC or %TSAT).

RECOMMENDATIONS

R39   People with anaemia of CKD who are receiving ESAs should be given iron therapy to maintain: (D(GPP))

- serum ferritin >200 µg/l
- transferrin saturation >20% (unless ferritin >800 µg/l)
- hypochromic red blood cells <6% (unless ferritin >800 µg/l)

Most patients will require 600–1,000 mg of iron for adults or equivalent doses for children, in a single or divided dose depending on the preparation. Patients with functional iron deficiency should be treated with intravenous iron. Peritoneal dialysis and non-dialysis patients who do not respond to oral iron will require intravenous iron. In appropriate circumstances, iron treatment can also be administered in the community.

R40   In non-dialysis patients with anaemia of CKD in whom there is evidence of absolute or functional iron deficiency, this should be corrected before deciding whether ESA therapy is necessary.   (D(GPP))

See 3.2.2 for the associated algorithm.

6.13 Treating iron deficiency: maintenance

6.13.1 Clinical introduction

See 6.12.1.

6.13.2 Methodological introduction

Because of the high number of retrieved studies in the literature search, these were grouped into:

- induction iron therapy for iron deficiency (both absolute and functional iron deficiency) and
- maintenance iron therapy for iron replete patients on epoetin

and thereafter further subgrouped into the various iron routes and frequencies of administration investigated. The seventeen studies included in the evidence statements were selected on the basis of evidence level hierarchy.

Two studies[240,241] did not meet quality criteria and were therefore excluded from the evidence statements.

Notable aspects of the evidence base were:

- Three studies were conducted in children.[242–244]
- Study durations ranged from 12 weeks to 18 months, which has implications on the time required to measure stability of treatment outcomes.

The GDG agreed that the following outcomes were priorities:

- epoetin dose
- efficacy/Hb response
- compliance
- patient preference
- side effects
- safety.

Following the first consultation on the guideline drafts, the GDG also considered additional retrospective studies[245–250] on the incidence of adverse events with intravenous iron. These papers did not report whether patients had previously had ESA therapy or not and because of potential confounding were not added as evidence statements but are discussed below under 'from evidence to recommendations' (see section 6.13.6).

6.13.3 Evidence statements

▷ Oral iron vs intravenous iron

Two RCTs[251,252] in adult dialysis patients with serum ferritin levels >100 µg/l compared i.v. and oral iron. One study[251] (n=52, all haemodialysis) administered 100 mg i.v. iron dextran twice a week and the other[252] (n=37, 15 haemodialysis and 19 peritoneal dialysis) administered 250 mg iron dextran fortnightly. Oral comparators were ferrous sulphate (200–325 mg tds) and iron polysaccharide (150 mg bd). Both studies found i.v. iron to be superior. In one study[251] haematocrit increased (p<0.05) and ESA dose fell (p<0.05); in the second study[252] haemoglobin increased (p<0.05) compared with those treated with oral iron. (**Level 1+**)

A study in predialysis patients[253] randomised patients with baseline ferritin levels of 47–155 µg/l to either oral ferrous sulphate 200 mg tds (n=23) or 300 mg intravenous iron sucrose. Over a follow-up period of 5.2 months, no significant difference in haemoglobin level or ESA requirement was observed. (**Level 1++**)

In a 29-day study with follow-up after 14 days[254] patients were randomised to epoetin and intermittent i.v. iron sucrose 200 mg bolus weekly (n=48) vs epoetin and ferrous sulphate (65 mg elemental iron) orally 3 times daily (n=48). Although the i.v. iron group had a greater increase in serum ferritin levels (p<0.0001), the rise in Hb from baseline was not statistically different between the two treatment groups. However, when patients were stratified by a baseline serum ferritin < or ≥100 µg/l, the i.v. iron group had a greater increase in Hb at follow-up compared with oral iron patients (p<0.05). Also, more patients in the i.v. iron group attained Hb >11.0 g/dl compared with the oral iron group (p=0.028) and the percentage change from baseline to follow-up for both Hb and ferritin was significantly greater for the i.v. iron group (p<0.0001). Mean treatment concordance assessed by tablet counts was lower in the oral iron group (85.5%) compared with the i.v. iron group (95.0%); no p-value was reported. GI side effects were more common in the oral iron group and taste disturbances in the i.v. iron group. No patient required discontinuation of iron treatment in either group. (**Level 1+**)

In a study conducted in peritoneal dialysis patients[255] comparing oral and intravenous iron using a crossover design, higher haematocrit levels (p=0.02) and lower ESA doses (p=0.008) were found with intravenous iron. Nine patients received oral ferrous sulphate 325 mg tds for 4 months followed by a single bolus infusion of 1 g iron dextran after a washout period of 1 month. (**Level 2+**)

One study conducted in children with TSAT>20%[242] randomised them to intravenous iron dextran or oral ferrous fumarate (n=35, all haemodialysis). Doses were based on weight; ferrous fumarate varied between 4 and 6 mg/kg/day, children <20 kg received 25 mg/week iron dextran, those weighing 20–40 kg received 50 mg/week and those >40 kg received 100 mg/week. After 16 weeks, no differences in ESA requirements or haemoglobin levels were found. (**Level 1+**)

▷ Intravenous iron studies in adults

Three observational studies in haemodialysis patients noted a reduction in ESA requirements with regular maintenance intravenous iron: p<0.0005,[256] p<0.05,[257] p<0.001.[258] One study[256] (n=116) used iron sucrose 100 mg post-haemodialysis. Another study[257] (n=24) used either a loading dose of 1g iron dextran given in divided doses over 10 consecutive dialyses followed by further boluses when TSAT fell below 20% or serum ferritin fell below 200 μg/l, or an initial pulse of iron dextran 300–500 mg followed by 25–100 mg every 1–2 weeks to maintain TSAT 30–50%. The third study[258] (n=396) maintained haemoglobin at a median level of 11.3 to 11.8 g/dl over a 24-month period. Patients with serum ferritin <500 μg/l were treated with concomitant i.v. iron sucrose regimen as follows: months 1–3, for ferritin <100 μg/l, 50 mg iron sucrose twice weekly, for ferritin 100–500 μg/l, 50 mg iron sucrose once weekly, months 4–9, for ferritin <100 μg/l, 50 mg iron sucrose twice weekly, for ferritin 100–500 ng/ml, iron sucrose dose depended on functional iron deficiency. Those with %HRC <5% were given 50 mg iron sucrose once weekly and those with %HRC >5%, 50 mg iron sucrose twice weekly. During months 10–24 those with ferritin <100 μg/l received 50 mg iron sucrose thrice weekly. Those with ferritin 100–500 μg/l received 50 mg iron sucrose once weekly if %HRC <2% (iron replete), or 50 mg iron sucrose twice weekly if %HRC 2–5%, or 50 mg iron sucrose thrice weekly if %HRC >5%. (**Level 2+ and Level 3**)

Another observational study in haemodialysis patients[259] stratified patients' responses to 20 mg intravenous iron saccharate given 3 times a week over a 6-month period by ferritin <100 μg/l (n=17) vs ≥100 <400 μg/l (n=16). Haemoglobin levels (p<0.0001) increased and ESA levels decreased (p<0.003) in all patients compared with baseline but there was no difference between groups. Four patients reported a metallic taste in association with iron but no other adverse events were reported. (**Level 2+**)

A further observational study[260] administered 100 mg intravenous ferric saccharate twice a month to 41 haemodialysis patients and 4 peritoneal dialysis patients who had been receiving ESAs for at least 6 months, and 11 haemodialysis patients who started ESA and intravenous iron simultaneously. In those previously on ESA, haematocrit levels were higher (p<0.05) and ESA doses lower (p<0.05) after 12 months. Those who started ESA and intravenous iron simultaneously had higher haematocrit levels (p<0.05) after 6 months of treatment. (**Level 2+**)

Four studies compared different intravenous iron dosing regimens.[261–264] In three studies conducted in haemodialysis patients the same total dose of iron was administered. One study[261] gave 400 mg saccharated ferric oxide in 10 divided doses either following 10 consecutive dialysis sessions (n=12) or weekly for 10 weeks (n=12). This study also included 11 subjects to whom iron was not administered. These patients had lower haemoglobin levels and greater ESA requirements compared with the iron–treated groups. The only difference in the iron treated groups was a lower ESA requirement compared with baseline (p<0.01) in those given sequential treatment after each dialysis. One study[262] gave a total of 600 mg iron dextran (n=43). Patients received either a single bolus dose, six divided doses of 100 mg following consecutive dialyses, or 100 mg/week for 6 weeks. No difference was observed in haemoglobin or ESA requirements with the different dosing regimens. (**Level 1+ and Level 2+**)

A further study in haemodialysis patients aiming for a target haemoglobin level of 11.8 g/dl compared three different iron dextran regimens.[263] A total dose infusion of 550–2000 mg was used in 14 patients, 12 patients received 500 mg/week as a bolus dose to a total of 400–1500 mg and 17 patients were given 100 mg/dialysis session to a total dose of 500–2100 mg. No differences in peak haematocrit or time to peak haematocrit were observed between groups. (**Level 1+**)

In peritoneal dialysis patients, one study[264] gave a total dose of intravenous ferric saccharate of 600 mg in divided doses with two different regimens using a crossover design (n=17). There was a greater increase in haematocrit levels in patients given 50 mg twice a week (p<0.05) compared with those given 100 mg/week. (**Level 1+**)

▷   Intravenous iron studies in children

In a 6-month study[243] (n=40) children below 16 years of age received epoetin to target Hct ≥30% and i.v. iron dextran administered as a maintenance dose of 1 mg/kg/week following a weight-based loading dose. This was compared with an as required intermittent weight-based course of 10 doses of iron dextran if Hct was <33%, ferritin <100 μg/l and/or TSAT <20%. Despite the higher cumulative dose in the intermittent group (p<0.001) the average epoetin dose was similar in both groups and Hb increased to 10 g/dl, with no difference between the 2 treatment groups. (**Level 1+**)

A double-blind RCT in children <16 years old receiving epoetin[244] randomised patients to concomitant treatment with eight consecutive intravenous infusions of either 1.5 mg/kg (n=24) or 3.0 mg/kg (n=32) of sodium ferric gluconate complex. Mean cumulative dose in the 1.5 mg/kg group was 431 ± 168 mg and 725 ± 202 mg in the 3.0 mg/kg group (p<0.0001). Although increases from baseline were found in both groups at 2- and 4-week evaluation time points after the last iron dose, no difference was found in Hb levels between the two groups. Responders were defined by Hb increase ≥1.0 g/dl. No difference was found between numbers of responders in either group. Epoetin dose remained unchanged in both treatment groups. (**Level 1+**)

▷   Intravenous iron safety studies

In a safety study, n=657 patients received 200 mg bolus injections of iron sucrose.[265] A total of 2,297 injections were administered, with some patients receiving multiple injections with a minimum of 1 week between injections. Mild and transient metallic taste was found for 412 injections and other adverse events for 57 injections. These were anaphylactoid reactions in seven patients, pain during injection in 31 patients, pain after injection in nine patients, with/without bruising, nausea/GI symptoms in three patients, lethargy in four patients, and light-headedness in three patients. (**Level 3**)

A cohort study[266] (n=32,566) sought to investigate if an apparent relationship between iron dosing and mortality was confounded by incomplete representation of iron dosing and morbidity over time. The study found doses of iron >1,000 mg over 6 months to be associated with increased risk of mortality compared with subjects not receiving iron using an adjusted proportional hazards analysis relating baseline iron dose to survival with a hazard ratio (HR) of 1.09 (95% CI 1.01–1.17). Those receiving >1800 mg of iron had HR 1.18 (95% CI 1.09–1.27). However, the association disappeared when the adjusted probability of dying in a particular month as a function of cumulative iron dose received during the previous 0 to 6 months, 6 to 12 months and 12 to 18 months was estimated. No significant association was found between mortality and any level of iron dosing >0 to >1,800 mg over 6 months. (**Level 2+**)

▷ Oral iron studies

One study[267] randomised iron replete patients to polysaccharide-iron complex 150 mg elemental iron twice daily (n=12) vs placebo (n=13) over 3 months with 2 months follow-up. No difference was found in Hct levels between the two groups. The same study also randomised iron deficient patients to either polysaccharide-iron complex 150 mg elemental iron twice daily (n=14) or placebo (n=10) over 3 months and 2 months follow-up. Those receiving iron had an increase in Hct levels (p<0.01) (**Level 1+**)

Another study[268] randomised patients to a number of different oral iron preparations containing a daily dose of 200 mg elemental iron, ferrous fumarate (Chromagen, n=12 and Tabron, n=11), ferrous sulphate (n=11) and iron-polysaccharide complex (n=12). Patients were also given various doses of daily ascorbic acid (750, 1,000, 0, 100 mg respectively) over 6 months. Hct levels increased with all preparations (Chromagen and ferrous sulphate, p<0.01; Tabron p<0.05), except for the iron-polysaccharide complex. In addition, Hct/epoetin ratio decreased (p<0.05) in the Tabron (ferrous fumarate) treatment group only. No differences were noted in compliance. (**Level 1+**)

6.13.4 Health economics methodological introduction

Six studies were appraised[269–274] and one study met quality criteria.[269] Three of the studies did not report unit costs, total costs or doses adequately[270,271,273] One study was excluded because of potential bias by physician adjustment of the epoetin dose in a before and after design.[272] One study[274] was excluded as cost-savings were not based on evidence.

6.13.5 Health economics evidence statements

One study found iron dextran did not reduce the average dose of ESA in 33 patients but improved the number of patients with 'successful treatment' (10 vs 27). Successful treatment was defined as Hct 33–36%, TSAT >20%, ferritin concentration of >100ng/ml and no blood administered except for acute blood loss. The study estimated the incremental cost effectiveness of iron dextran to be $41.61 (US$, 1998) per successful treatment.[269] No sensitivity analysis was performed.

6.13.6 From evidence to recommendations

The published evidence was very limited in peritoneal dialysis and predialysis patients. It did not provide data to allow the GDG to specify a test dose of iron in the recommendations, nor a route or frequency of administration.

Caution is required because of the potential side-effect profile (particularly anaphylaxis) when administering both test and maintenance doses of iron. The GDG considered additional retrospective studies of adverse events in patients receiving intravenous iron to inform the recommendations:

- Baillie et al[245] investigated tens of millions of 100mg dose equivalents (the exact sample size is not given in the paper) from the American Food and Drug Administration (FDA) 'freedom of information surveillance database'. They considered all adverse events between January 1997 and September 2002 and found rates per million 100mg dose equivalents of 29.2 for iron dextran, 10.5 for sodium ferric gluconate and 4.2 for iron sucrose (which had the lowest rates for all clinical categories of adverse event).
- Chertow et al[246,247] investigated 30,063,800 doses in FDA data from 2001 to 2003 and found significantly lower rates among people who received sodium ferric gluconate or iron sucrose, compared with those who received higher molecular weight iron dextran. Rates of 'life-threatening' events per million doses were 11.3 for higher molecular weight iron dextran, 3.3 for lower molecular weight iron dextran, 0.9 for sodium ferric gluconate, and 0.6 for iron sucrose.
- Fishbane et al[248] investigated all patients (n=573) receiving intravenous iron dextran at any of four USA haemodialysis centres between July 1993 and June 1995 and found 27 patients (4.7%) had related adverse events. History of drug allergy (OR 2.4, p=0.03) and multiple drug allergy (OR 5.5, p<0.001) were found to be significant risk factors for adverse events.
- Fletes et al[249] investigated the Fresenius Medical Care North America (FMCNA) clinical variance reports from October 1998 to March 1999 for iron dextran only and found an adverse event rate of 196.1 per million doses. The study reported higher rates in patients receiving higher molecular weight iron dextran, but this was not statistically significant.
- Walters and van Wyck[250] investigated 1,066,099 doses of intravenous iron dextran from the Gambro Healthcare US database between January 1999 and April 2000. They found a rate of 316.1 adverse events per million doses for all severities, and reported in detail on seven patients who had adverse events requiring resuscitation, all of whom were receiving test doses or first therapeutic doses. Significance testing to compare molecular weights of iron dextran was only reported for these seven patients.

Adverse event rates for intravenous iron are very low for both preparations in use in the UK (circa 3.3 events per million doses for low molecular weight iron dextran, and 0.6 per million doses for iron sucrose), and the GDG therefore did not distinguish between them in the recommendation.

The GDG acknowledged the cost-effectiveness evidence of predialysis anaemia treatments is limited as there is little data to make comparisons to alternative treatments and insufficient effectiveness data of patient benefit such as quality of life. The GDG noted that collecting quality of life data that could be converted into utility scores and resource data in all future randomised controlled trials would be useful, especially in predialysis patients.

RECOMMENDATION

R41   Once ferritin >200 µg/l and HRC <6% or TSAT >20%, people with anaemia of CKD who are receiving ESAs should be given maintenance iron. The dosing regimen will depend on modality, for example haemodialysis patients will require the equivalent of 50–60 mg intravenous iron per week (or an equivalent dose in children of 1 mg/kg/week). Peritoneal dialysis and non-dialysis patients who do not respond to oral iron will require intravenous iron.   **(D(GPP))**

See 3.2.2 for the associated algorithm.

6.14 ESAs: monitoring iron status during treatment

6.14.1 Clinical introduction

Measurement of ferritin together with %HRC or %TSAT provides an indication of iron stores and availability of iron for erythropoiesis. We know that in patients with anaemia associated with CKD who are under treatment with ESAs, an adequate supply of iron is essential for effective erythropoiesis and cost-efficient use of ESAs. We also know that too much iron may expose patients to risk of infectious complications and may also increase cardiovascular risk through oxidative stress. What then are the most desirable levels of these parameters of iron status to be maintained during treatment with ESAs?

6.14.2 Clinical methodological introduction

A literature search identified four studies consisting of a RCT,[77] a cohort study,[275] a prospective longitudinal study[258] and a prospective longitudinal study in children.[276]

One study[277] did not meet quality criteria and was therefore excluded from the evidence statements.

Notable aspects of the evidence base were:

- In the study comparing TSAT 20–30% and 30–50%,[77] achieved TSAT levels were 27.6% and 32.6% in the respective groups at the end of the 6-month study period.

6.14.3 Clinical evidence statements

▷   Serum ferritin

Haemodialysis patients

Intravenous iron supplementation which led to an increase in mean ferritin to 395 ± 206 mg/100 ml (p-value not given) in children aged 10–17 years (n=8) lead to an increase in the Hb (p=0.0117) and Hct (p=0.0024), despite a fall in epoetin dose from 6,500 U to 6,150 U with no side effects noted, particularly hypertension.[276] (**Level 3**)

In a 24-month study (n=396)[258] Hb was maintained at a median level of 11.3 to 11.8 g/dl and median epoetin dose decreased to 72 (inter-quartile range 33–134) (p<0.001) when compared with baseline, when patients with serum ferritin <500 ng/ml were treated with concomitant i.v. iron sucrose regimen. (**Level 3+**)

▷ Transferrin saturation (TSAT)

Haemodialysis patients

In a study comparing the effects of TSAT 20–30% vs 30–50% on epoetin dose required to maintain Hb 9.5–12.0 g/dl, epoetin dose progressively decreased in the TSAT 30–50% group, with ~40% dose reduction in months 4, 5 and 6 when compared with the 20–30% group (p=0.0038). This change in epoetin dose was independent of baseline dose in both the TSAT 30–50% group and TSAT 20–30% group.[77] (**Level 1+**)

▷ Percentage of hypochromic red cells (%HRC)

Haemodialysis patients

In an 8-week study whereby patients stratified by baseline %HRC 0–3%, 4–9% and ≥10% received a fixed epoetin dose and i.v. iron saccharate 200 mg once weekly up to serum ferritin 250 µg/l, although mean Hb and ferritin levels significantly increased in all 3 groups (P≤0.001 for all), mean Hb increase was greater with increasing %HRC at baseline (p=0.02). In addition the proportion of patients with >1 g/dl increase in Hb was greater as %HRC at baseline increased (p=0.02).[275] (**Level 2+**)

6.14.4 Health economic methodological introduction

Three studies were appraised[77,273,278] and two met quality criteria.[77,278] The study that did not meet quality criteria estimated cost-savings based on average reduced EPO dosages.[273] However, with no inclusion of the prices used, the costing was not sufficiently transparent to warrant inclusion.

An American study estimated the cost-savings per patient per year over a 6-month period while maintaining TSAT between 30 and 50% vs 20 to 30% using maintenance intravenous iron dextran.[77]

One American study was a cost analysis of ESAs using percent reduction of urea (PRU) as an index of dialysis adequacy and transferrin saturation as a measure of iron stores. The study investigated two comparisons: the total dose of ESA received during the 4-week study by the 20 participants with the highest transferrin saturation to the 20 participants with the lowest transferrin saturation, and the total dose of ESA administered during the 4-week study to the 20 patients with the highest PRU to the 20 participants with the lowest PRU.[278]

6.14.5 Health economic evidence statements

The study estimated intravenous iron dextran saves approximately $109 per month or $1,308 per year per patient when maintaining the TSAT between 30 and 50% (n=23) (vs 20 to 30% in control group; n=19).[77] Cost difference between the intervention and control group was statistically significant by the third month of study and remained significant until the end of the study at 6 months (p<0.02).[77]

At $10 per 1,000 units of ESA, it costs $45 (10.2%) more per month per patient in the 20 patients with the lowest transferrin saturation compared with the 20 patients with the highest transferrin saturation.[278]

6.14.6 From evidence to recommendations

The GDG agreed that there was very little long-term effectiveness data to determine the most appropriate maintenance levels. The GDG based their recommendation on the European Best Practice Guidelines.[279]

RECOMMENDATIONS

R42   Patients receiving ESA maintenance therapy should be given iron supplements to keep their:

- serum ferritin between 200 and 500 µg/l in both haemodialysis patients and   (D)
  non-haemodialysis patients, **and either**
  - the transferrin saturation level above 20% (unless ferritin
    > 800 µg/l) **or**   (B)
  - percentage hypochromic red cells (%HRC) less than 6% (unless ferritin
    > 800 µg/l).   (D(GPP))

In practice it is likely this will require intravenous iron.

7 | Monitoring treatment of anaemia of CKD

7.1 Monitoring iron status

7.1.1 Clinical introduction

Monitoring of iron status should be aimed at ensuring that patients undergoing treatment with ESAs maintain levels of iron that ensure maximally effective erythropoiesis. The frequency of monitoring must take account of the stage of anaemia treatment, ie initial correction of anaemia or maintenance of target range of haemoglobin, the frequency and mode of iron supplementation, CKD status (haemodialysis patients have an unavoidable loss of iron through the dialysis process), clinical situations likely to result in depletion of iron stores such as bleeding and surgery, clinical situations likely to result in misinterpretation of iron parameters (for example, co-existent infection leads to falsely elevated ferritin levels and depressed %TSAT), and pre-existing iron-overload states. The frequency of monitoring may also be dictated by the availability of the patient and by trend analysis of changes in iron status over time.

7.1.2 Methodological introduction

A comprehensive literature search identified a cohort study.[257]

A comprehensive literature search did not identify any studies that were suitable to address the economic aspects of this section, therefore no health economic evidence statements are given.

7.1.3 Evidence statements

▷ Monitoring after intermittent iron dosing

Haemodialysis patients

Table 7.1 Time profile of intermittent i.v. iron dextran dosing regimen (n=14) (Level 2)

Treatment with 1,000 mg iron dextran over 10 doses	T=0	T=3 days	Time averaged value over 4 months after completion (trapezoid method)
TSAT (%)	20.6 ± 2.0 (range 15–37)	93 ± 6 (range 63–134)	30.1
	T=0	T=2 months (peak value)	
Ferritin (ng/ml)	197 ± 31 (range 27–424)	351	
	T=0	T=3 months	T=4 months
TIBC (µg/ml)	210 ± 7 (166–246)	180 ± 7	192 ± 11

▷ Monitoring after single iron dose

Haemodialysis patients

Table 7.2 Time profile of single dose i.v. iron dextran 50 mg or 100 mg (n=16) **(Level 2+)**		
	T=0	**Time averaged over 2 weeks**
TSAT (%)	Mean 34.6 ± 3.1 (n=16)	• 35.5 for 50 mg group (n=8) • 36.7 for 100 mg group (n=8)
	T=0	
Ferritin (ng/ml)	231 ± 29 (n=16)	T=1 week, 297 ± 44 (n=16) T=2 weeks, 276 ± 35 (n=16)
	T=0	**Time averaged over 2 weeks**
TIBC (µg/ml)	Not reported	No change (data not reported)

7.1.4 From evidence to recommendations

The GDG agreed on a range of possible intervals for iron stores monitoring, which will allow practice to be tailored to the individual patient and to local systems. It is clear from the evidence that monitoring soon after intravenous iron is not helpful, and the GDG felt that a minimum time elapsed of 1 week would be appropriate.

RECOMMENDATIONS

R43   People with anaemia of CKD should not have iron levels checked earlier than 1 week after receiving intravenous iron. The length of time to monitoring of iron status is dependant on the product used and the amount of iron given.   (C)

R44   Routine monitoring of iron stores should be at intervals of 4 weeks to 3 months.   (D(GPP))

7.2 Monitoring haemoglobin levels

7.2.1 Clinical introduction

The initial step in clinical management of the CKD patient maintained in an anaemia programme must be the acquisition of laboratory and treatment data at specified intervals. The frequency of acquisition of data has been driven by anaemia treatment algorithms and decision matrices designed to achieve the required rate of rise of haemoglobin during the correction phase, and the desired haemoglobin level during the maintenance phase. However, the effectiveness of such algorithms and decision matrices is difficult to evaluate because there is a lack of published clinical outcomes related to their use. Furthermore, there is inherent variability in haemoglobin levels within a given population, and there are several components of this variability. One component is population or interpatient variability. Biological variability is found with nearly all laboratory measurements and in the case of haemoglobin levels in patients with CKD multiple factors contribute including gender and race, environmental factors, assay or sampling differences, the patient's state of hydration and other related physiological determinants. Another component of haemoglobin level variability is individual or intraindividual variability. Here there is variation with repeated measurements over time in the same individual. Again there are multiple factors contributing to this variability including seasonal variations, sampling methods, comorbid conditions such as nutritional status, inflammation, gastrointestinal bleeding, and bone marrow fibrosis. Two major factors are under control of the anaemia management team: ESA and iron therapy, and these are also determinants of haemoglobin level and factors in population variability. The physiological characteristics of erythropoiesis are such that there is a time required for the bone marrow to react to changing ESA stimulus and that reaction time varies widely among patients with CKD, ranging from a few weeks to a few months. It requires 1 to 2 months to induce red blood cell production and 1 to 3 months after removal of ESA stimulus for patients to experience turnover of red blood cells to cease production. Data from a 1-year study demonstrates that haemoglobin levels may change from less than 11 g/dl to greater than 12 g/dl (or vice versa) in more than 28% of patients.[212] Haemoglobin synthesis, red blood cell production and destruction are not processes that can be controlled instantaneously and haemoglobin level undershooting or overshooting should be expected when health professionals react to single haemoglobin values. We should therefore react to trends in haemoglobin levels but how frequently should the haemoglobin level be monitored to determine the trend?

7.2.2 Methodological introduction

A comprehensive literature search did not identify any studies that were suitable to address the clinical or economic aspects of this section, therefore no evidence statements are given.

7.2.3 From evidence to recommendations

Monitoring is part of care in ESA induction and maintenance, including consideration of the rate of haemoglobin change. The GDG felt that a range of intervals would allow monitoring to be tailored to the patient and the local systems, and agreed on 2–4 weeks in induction and 1–3 months in maintenance.

RECOMMENDATION

R45 In people with anaemia of CKD, haemoglobin should be monitored:
- every 2–4 weeks in the induction phase of ESA therapy
- every 1–3 months in the maintenance phase of ESA therapy
- more actively after an ESA dose adjustment
- in a clinical setting chosen in discussion with the patient, taking into consideration their convenience and local healthcare systems. (D(GPP))

7.3 Detecting ESA resistance

7.3.1 Clinical introduction

The physiological characteristics of erythropoiesis are such that there is a time required for the bone marrow to react to ESA stimulus and that reaction time varies widely among patients with CKD, ranging from a few weeks to a few months. The magnitude of reaction to ESA stimulus is also variable. In determining resistance to ESA therapy it is important to distinguish between true resistance, a lack of bone marrow response to ESA therapy, and apparent resistance where increased red cell destruction or red cell loss offsets ESA stimulated red cell production. It is also important to determine a dose threshold of ESA above which resistance to therapy is defined and a duration of therapy beyond which resistance to therapy should be suspected.

7.3.2 Methodological introduction

A literature search identified a case series[280] and a cohort study.[281]

Five studies[282–286] did not meet quality criteria and were therefore excluded from the evidence statements.

A comprehensive literature search did not identify any studies that were suitable to address the economic aspects of this section, therefore no evidence statements are given.

7.3.3 Evidence statements

▷ Pure red cell aplasia (PRCA)

Haemodialysis patients

In a study of patients predominantly receiving subcutaneous epoetin alfa, serum from all epoetin-treated patients (n=13) inhibited growth of erythroid cells and addition of epoetin to their serum samples reversed inhibitory effects. Also serum from all patients was shown to bind to epoetin and Scatchard analysis suggested presence of homogeneous binding sites.[280] (**Level 3**)

▷ Aluminium toxicity

Haemodialysis patients

In a study conducted to maintain Hct 30% (Hb ~10 g/dl), where patients were divided into 2 groups on the basis of response to epoetin treatment, the poor responders received a higher epoetin dose ($p<0.05$), yet had lower Hb and Hct levels (both $p<0.001$). Of the haematological parameters investigated, basal aluminium and aluminium levels following challenge with desferrioxamine were higher in the poor responders (both $p<0.01$). In addition, mean corpuscular volume showed inverse correlation with basal aluminium (data not provided), post-desferrioxamine aluminium ($r=-0.617$, $p=0.005$) and change in aluminium levels ($r=-0.711$, $p<0.001$) in the poor responders. In the good responders, mean corpuscular volume only showed correlation with change in aluminium levels ($r=-0.476$, $p=0.03$).[281] (**Level 2+**)

7.3.4 From evidence to recommendations

In considering when resistance to ESAs should be suspected and what conditions lead to ESA resistance, the GDG reviewed evidence on two outcomes, PRCA and aluminium toxicity.

The GDG considered the definition of resistance and agreed on the definition suggested by the *Revised European best practice guidelines for the management of anaemia in patients with chronic renal failure.*[287] It was agreed to suspect resistance when a patient does not achieve the target Hb level after receiving an epoetin dose more than 300 U/kg/week s.c. (approximately 20,000 units/week) or equivalent or 1.5 mg/kg darbepoetin alfa s.c. or i.v. (approximately 100 mg/week) or has a continued need for the administration of high doses of ESAs to maintain the target Hb level.[287] It was noted that 300 U/kg/week is used as this value is two standard deviations above the mean value used. The GDG considered that resistance should be suspected after 3 months of failure to respond to ESAs, after exclusion of other causes of a temporary lack of response (eg intercurrent illness or other causes of chronic bleeding).

With regards to conditions that lead to ESA resistance the GDG reviewed evidence on PRCA. The GDG agreed their working definition of PRCA to be the presence of a low reticulocyte count, together with anaemia and the presence of neutralising antibodies. The GDG considered PRCA to be confirmed where anti-erythropoietin antibodies are present (as shown by an appropriate laboratory assay) and there was a lack of pro-erythroid progenitor cells in the bone marrow. The GDG noted that PRCA can be induced by other causes aside from sensitisation to erythropoietin. This has since been addressed by using a fluoro-resin coating, which forms a barrier between the rubber stopper and erythropoietin in some pre-filled syringes. The evidence presented specifically addressed PRCA induced by sensitisation to erythropoietin and demonstrated that the inhibition of the erythroid cells was correlated with the presence of anti-erythropoietin antibodies.[280]

The GDG noted that the issue of aluminium toxicity was of clinical importance but the incidence is now very rare. The GDG noted that there was a current source of aluminium from the responsible use of aluminium hydroxide capsules (Alu-caps, used as phosphate binders to reduce the absorption of dietary phosphate). However, it was considered unlikely that the use of Alu-caps would lead to aluminium toxicity. The issue of toxicity originally stemmed from a lack of water purity which has improved. It was noted that the trial[281] did not report either the use of aluminium-based phosphate binders or whether any water purification system was being used. The GDG noted that aluminium levels are routinely measured in their haemodialysis patients but that the need to continue doing so was under question.

RECOMMENDATIONS

R46   After other causes of anaemia, such as intercurrent illness or chronic blood loss have been excluded, people with anaemia of CKD should be considered resistant to ESAs when:

- an aspirational Hb range is not achieved despite treatment with ≥300 IU/kg/week of subcutaneous epoetin or ≥450 IU/kg/week of intravenous epoetin or 1.5 μg/kg/week of darbepoetin, or
- there is a continued need for the administration of high doses of ESAs to maintain the aspirational Hb range.   (D(GPP))

R47   In people with CKD, pure red cell aplasia (PRCA) is indicated by a low reticulocyte count, together with anaemia and the presence of neutralising antibodies. The GDG considered that PRCA should be confirmed when anti-erythropoietin antibodies are present and there is a lack of pro-erythroid progenitor cells in the bone marrow.   (D)

R48   In people with anaemia of CKD, aluminium toxicity should be considered as a potential cause of a reduced response to ESAs after other causes such as intercurrent illness and chronic blood loss have been excluded.   (C)

See 3.2.4 for the associated algorithm.

7.4   Managing ESA resistance

7.4.1   Clinical introduction

Management of ESA resistance will clearly depend on the underlying cause. The Netherlands Cooperative Study on Adequacy of Dialysis (NECOSAD-2) identified an incidence of inadequate ESA response of 16.7 per 1,000 patients years on ESA while on dialysis.[288] Fifty-seven of 1,677 patients with incident end stage renal disease in the NECOSAD-2 study had an inadequate ESA response. Table 7.3 shows the various causes identified.

Table 7.3 Possible causes for ESA resistance from the NECOSAD-2 study (n=57)			
Causes for inadequate ESA response	**Number***	**Causes for inadequate ESA response**	**Number***
Infection/inflammation	41	Haemolysis	0
Blood loss	16	Pure red cell aplasia	1
Hyperparathyroidism/aluminium toxicity	10	Malignancy	7
Haemoglobinopathy	2	Graft/shunt problems	14
Folate/vitamin B12 deficiency	1	Operation	8
Multiple myeloma/myelofibrosis/ myelodysplastic syndrome	6	Suspected noncompliance	9
Malnutrition	5	Medication (≥bone marrow suppress)	4
Inadequate dialysis	2	Unknown	2

*Some patients fell into more than one category (ie there was more than one possible cause for their inadequate ESA response).

7.4.2   Methodological introduction

The literature search identified three studies: a 2-part study with a prospective cohort group and a subsequent before and after study in a subgroup,[289] a retrospective case series[290] and a before and after study.[291]

A comprehensive literature search did not identify any studies that were suitable to address the economic aspects of this section, therefore no evidence statements are given.

7.4.3 Evidence statements

▷ Treatment of aluminium toxicity with desferrioxamine

Dialysis patients

Patients receiving epoetin with no concurrent or prior treatment for aluminium toxicity (n=5) had a low mean rise of Hb above baseline and did not achieve target Hb 9 g/dl over 20 weeks, unlike the control groups with treatment prior to the study (n=4) (p<0.05) and no aluminium toxicity (n=8) (p<0.05), which reached target Hb within 12 weeks of the study.[289] This was supported by the correlation between baseline serum aluminium levels and the mean rise of Hb (r=−0.51, p=0.03) and between Hb rise during epoetin therapy and aluminium increment following challenge with desferrioxamine. (**Level 2+**)

In addition, concurrent treatment with desferrioxamine in this group led to a mean Hb rise when compared with previous treatment with epoetin only (p<0.01).[289] (**Level 3**)

▷ Reduced T-cell production of inflammatory markers TNF-α and IFN-γ with low dose pentoxifylline

Patient population not specified

Hb levels in poor responders to epoetin (n=12) significantly improved after 4 months treatment with low dose pentoxifylline (p=0.0001). This was associated with a decrease in TNF-α (p=0.0007) and IFN-γ (p=0.0002) production 6–8 weeks following pentoxifylline therapy, and no change in white blood cell production after 4 months. This suggestive evidence was supported by a correlation between change in Hb and TNF-α production (r_s=0.7145, p=0.0118), however, no correlation was found between change in Hb and IFN-γ (r_s=0.4406, p=0.1542).[291] (**Level 3**)

▷ Treatment of ESA-induced pure red cell aplasia (PRCA) with immunosuppressants/immunoglobulins/kidney transplant

Not on dialysis, haemodialysis and peritoneal dialysis patients

In a group of patients with epoetin-induced PRCA (n=43 epoetin alfa ± epoetin beta or darbepoetin and n=4 epoetin beta exclusively), 37 patients received treatment which consisted of one treatment (n=26), two consecutive treatment regimens (n=10) or five different regimens (n=1). Of these, 29 patients recovered (ie reticulocyte counts >20,000/µl and not requiring red cell transfusions), however, no patient was challenged with ESA. As the treatments are not comparable for superiority, the data from the study is presented in the Table 7.4.

Table 7.4 Summary data from Verhelst (2004)[290] (Level 3)

PRCA treatment	n	Number of patients who recovered	Time before recovery (months)	Follow-up (months)
Corticosteroids alone (n=14) ± high dose i.v. immunoglobulins	18	10 (56%)	1[†], 2[†], 2[†], 3[†], 3[†], 3[†], 3[†], 3[†], 6[†], 18[†]	3, 3, 3, 3, 5[†], 13[†], 20, 30[†]
High dose i.v. immunoglobulins alone	9	1 (11%)	3[†]	3, 3, 4, 4, 4, 9, 10[†], 19
Corticosteroids + cyclophosphamide	8	7 (87%)	1[†], 2, 2, 3[†], 4, 5, 7	3
Ciclosporin	6	4 (67%)	1[†], 1[†], 1[†], 1	3, 9[†]
Kidney transplant*	6	6 (100%)	<1[†], <1[†], <1[†], <1[†], <1, <1	–
Antibodies to CD20	2	0	–	3[†], 3
Corticosteroids + high dose i.v. immunoglobulins + plasma exchange	1	1 (100%)	3[†]	–
Mycophenolate motefil	1	0	–	12

Note: for patients who did not recover, follow-up was length of time between start of treatment and last visit or start of new treatment.
[†]Received only 1 kind of treatment. * Received induction treatment followed by triple immunosuppressive therapy.

7.4.4 From evidence to recommendations

When considering how ESA resistance should be managed the GDG reviewed evidence on three outcomes, aluminium toxicity, markers of inflammation and the treatment of PRCA.

The GDG noted that with regard to treating aluminium toxicity that desferrioxamine was considered the treatment of choice. If aluminium toxicity was suspected, a patient should be administered a bolus of desferrioxamine and the amount of aluminium flushed into the blood stream determined. Treatment with desferrioxamine should be administered until aluminium toxicity is no longer present. The GDG noted that it was rare to find patients with toxic levels of aluminium and that this should be considered a special circumstance that would be most likely to occur in haemodialysis patients managed by renal physicians.

With regard to inflammatory markers, the GDG reviewed one study that suggested that in poor responders to ESAs, treatment with low-dose pentoxifylline reduced the production of inflammatory markers (TNF-α and IFN-γ) by T-cells.[291] However, the GDG cautioned that this was an academic scientific study that, although interesting, did not reflect current clinical practice and noted that pentoxifylline was not licensed for this use. The GDG felt that clinical trials were needed to support this data.

The GDG reviewed evidence on the treatment of ESA-mediated PRCA. The GDG felt this was a specialised area with few annual cases. Because of this, the GDG acknowledged that the treatment of this condition was not fully established and that the most up-to-date information was available online and was written by the PRCA Global Scientific Advisory Board (GSAB: www.prcaforum.com/treatment.php) [292] and this should be accessed to determine the current best practice to treat this condition. The GDG noted that immunosuppressive therapies have been shown to reverse antibody-mediated PRCA. However, it was noted that the total number of patients with this condition was so small that they felt unable to recommend this treatment. The GDG noted that the GSAB suggested ciclosporin as the treatment of choice.

RECOMMENDATIONS

R49   In haemodialysis patients with anaemia of CKD in whom aluminium toxicity is suspected, a desferrioxamine test should be performed and the patient's management reviewed accordingly.   (C)

R50   ESA-induced PRCA should be managed in accordance with current best practice. Specialist referral should be considered.

Note: current best practice for this rare condition is available from the PRCA Global Scientific Advisory Board (GSAB: www.prcaforum.com/treatment.php).

See section 3.2.4 for the associated algorithm.

8 | Research recommendations

The Guideline Development Group has made the following recommendations for research, on the basis of its review of the evidence. The Group regards these recommendations as the most important research areas to improve NICE guidance and patient care in the future.

Intravenous iron in children

A prospective study of adequate duration of i.v. iron preparations in children with anaemia of CKD, including safety, dosing and efficacy outcomes.

▷ Why this is important

There is very little evidence relating to anaemia of CKD in children. It is known that there is a range of iron levels for adults outside which adverse outcomes become more likely and this helps guide monitoring and treatment adjustment over anaemia correction and maintenance. In children, there is likely to be much greater variation between individuals.

Trials of ESAs in children

Trials of ESAs in children with anaemia of CKD (including darbepoetin, which is currently unlicensed in children younger than 12 years), including safety, dosing and efficacy outcomes.

▷ Why this is important

As above, there is very little evidence relating to anaemia of CKD in children. ESAs are a key therapy and therefore more data are needed in order to define suitable treatment regimens.

Haemoglobin levels in older people

An observational study of Hb levels and adverse outcomes in older people.

▷ Why this is important

Evidence suggests that anaemia due to reduced erythropoiesis occurs even in early stages of CKD. This may be undetected, and is associated with adverse outcomes in older people. A better understanding of the haemoglobin levels associated with adverse outcomes in older people would enable improved detection of anaemia of CKD and reduction of risk.

ESA tolerance test

A trial of an ESA tolerance test including collection of data on ESA regimens and Hb levels achieved.

▷ Why this is important

A better understanding of the practical impact of ESA tolerance testing on treatment and outcomes would clarify whether such tests are useful, particularly in terms of tailoring ESAs and optimal Hb levels for individual patients depending on their response.

Iron levels in predialysis patients

An RCT to assess Hb level as an outcome in predialysis patients treated to serum ferritin levels <200 µg/l vs those treated to 300–500 µg/l.

▷ Why this is important

The ferritin level up to which predialysis patients should be treated to achieve acceptable Hb (and at which ESAs are considered if Hb is still inadequate) is not well addressed in the evidence base.

Implementation of management algorithm

An observational study of patient management in line with the initial management and maintenance algorithms given in this guideline, with the aim of formally piloting and validating them, or providing evidence for amendments when the guideline is updated.

▷ Why this is important

Protocols and prescribing algorithms for ESAs are in use, including computerised decision support systems. Some of these have been piloted and validated, and it is important that the NICE guideline's algorithms match this standard to provide additional support at the broader scale of management strategies.

Other potential research topics

Optimal Hb levels to be achieved with ESAs in children with ACKD.

Are the same levels of serum ferritin, %HRC and %TSAT that define functional iron deficiency in dialysis patients applicable to the predialysis population?

The value of endogenous erythropoietin testing in the diagnosis of anaemia associated with CKD.

Which patients would most benefit from ESA therapy in the wider CKD population?

Does the co-administration of ESAs with physiological doses of androgens reduce the dose of ESA administered?

Appendix A: Evidence-based clinical questions and literature searches

Question ID	Question wording	Study type filters used	Databases and years
PROG1	In patients with chronic kidney disease, what haemoglobin (Hb) / haematocrit levels are associated with adverse outcomes and what are the effects of a) age b) gender c) ethnicity?	All study types	Medline 1966–2005 Embase 1980–2005 Cochrane 1800–2005 Cinahl 1982–2005
DIAG1	In patients with chronic kidney disease, what is the association between glomerular filtration rate (GFR) and haemoglobin levels in a) diabetic and b) non-diabetic patients?	All study types	Medline 1966–2005 Embase 1980–2005 Cochrane 1800–2005 Cinahl 1982–2005
DTEST2	What are the best tests, or combination of tests, to determine iron status in patients with chronic kidney disease?	Diagnosis	Medline 1966–2005 Embase 1980–2005 Cochrane 1800–2005 Cinahl 1982–2005
DTEST1	What is the role of erythropoietin testing in the assessment of anaemia in patients with chronic kidney disease?	All study types	Medline 1966–2005 Embase 1980–2005 Cochrane 1800–2005 Cinahl 1982–2005
MGTFE1	Up to what levels of serum ferritin, percentage transferrin saturation and percentage hypochromic red cells should patients with ACKD be treated with iron without adverse events?	Systematic reviews, RCTs and comparative studies	Medline 1966–2005 Embase 1980–2005 Cochrane 1800–2005 Cinahl 1982–2005
MGTFE2	In patients with ACKD what, if any, are the serum ferritin, transferrin saturation and percentage hypochromic red cells thresholds for commencing treatment with ESAs?	Systematic reviews, RCTs and comparative studies	Medline 1966–2005 Embase 1980–2005 Cochrane 1800–2005 Cinahl 1982–2005
MGTFE3	In patients with ACKD what, if any, are the optimal serum ferritin, transferrin saturation and percentage hypochromic red cells levels to be maintained during treatment with ESAs?	Systematic reviews, RCTs and comparative studies	Medline 1966–2005 Embase 1980–2005 Cochrane 1800–2005 Cinahl 1982–2005
MGTN1	What is the benefit of vitamin C, vitamin E, folic acid, carnitine or glutathione supplementation in the treatment of anaemia due to chronic kidney disease?	Systematic reviews and RCTs	Medline 1966–2005 Embase 1980–2005 Cochrane 1800–2005 Cinahl 1982–2005
MGTN2	What is the benefit of androgens in the treatment of anaemia due to chronic kidney disease?	Systematic reviews and RCTs	Medline 1966–2005 Embase 1980–2005 Cochrane 1800–2005 Cinahl 1982–2005

continued

Evidence-based clinical questions and literature searches – *continued*

Question ID	Question wording	Study type filters used	Databases and years
HYP1	When does treating hyperparathyroidism improve the management of anaemia caused by chronic kidney disease?	All study types	Medline 1966–2005 Embase 1980–2005 Cochrane 1800–2005 Cinahl 1982–2005
PAT1	What are the patient preferences and experiences when receiving ESAs for the treatment of ACKD?	All study types	Medline 1966–2005 Embase 1980–2005 Cochrane 1800–2005 Cinahl 1982–2005 BNI 1985–2005
PAT2	Is the effectiveness of anaemia management of CKD improved by patient education programmes?	All study types	Medline 1966–2005 Embase 1980–2005 Cochrane 1800–2005 Cinahl 1982–2005 BNI 1985–2005 PsycInfo 1806–2005
MGTHB1	What haemoglobin range should be maintained during anaemia treatment in CKD?	Systematic reviews, RCTs and comparative studies	Medline 1966–2005 Embase 1980–2005 Cochrane 1800–2005 Cinahl 1982–2005
MGTHB2	In patients with chronic kidney disease what are the risks and benefits of early vs deferred correction of anaemia?	Systematic reviews and RCTs	Medline 1966–2005 Embase 1980–2005 Cochrane 1800–2005 Cinahl 1982–2005
TXFE1	What is the most effective and safest dose, frequency, preparation and route of administration of iron in ACKD patients with functional iron deficiency prior to ESA treatment?	Systematic reviews and RCTs	Medline 1966–2005 Embase 1980–2005 Cochrane 1800–2005 Cinahl 1982–2005
TXFE2	What is the most effective and safest dose, frequency, preparation and route of administration of iron in ACKD patients with functional iron deficiency receiving ESA treatment?	Systematic reviews and RCTs	Medline 1966–2005 Embase 1980–2005 Cochrane 1800–2005 Cinahl 1982–2005
TXEF1	In patients with ACKD what are the benefits and risks of correcting anaemia with epoetin alfa compared to epoetin beta in reducing morbidity and mortality and improving quality of life?	Systematic reviews, RCTs and comparative studies	Medline 1966–2005 Embase 1980–2005 Cochrane 1800–2005 Cinahl 1982–2005
TXEF2	In patients with ACKD what are the benefits and risks of correcting anaemia with epoetin alfa compared to darbepoetin in reducing morbidity and mortality and improving quality of life?	Systematic reviews, RCTs and comparative studies	Medline 1966–2005 Embase 1980–2005 Cochrane 1800–2005 Cinahl 1982–2005
TXEF3	In patients with ACKD what are the benefits and risks of correcting anaemia with epoetin beta compared to darbepoetin in reducing morbidity and mortality and improving quality of life?	Systematic reviews, RCTs and comparative studies	Medline 1966–2005 Embase 1980–2005 Cochrane 1800–2005 Cinahl 1982–2005
TXEF4	In patients with ACKD what are the benefits and risks of correcting anaemia with ESAs compared to placebo or no treatment in reducing morbidity and mortality and improving quality of life?	Systematic reviews, RCTs and comparative studies	Medline 1966–2005 Embase 1980–2005 Cochrane 1800–2005 Cinahl 1982–2005

continued

Evidence-based clinical questions and literature searches – *continued*

Question ID	Question wording	Study type filters used	Databases and years
MGTE1	Which iron replete patients with ACKD should receive ESAs?	Systematic reviews, RCTs and comparative studies	Medline 1966–2005 Embase 1980–2005 Cochrane 1800–2005 Cinahl 1982–2005
TXEF5	In patients with ACKD what are the benefits and risks of correcting anaemia with blood transfusions in reducing morbidity and mortality and improving quality of life?	Systematic reviews, RCTs and comparative studies	Medline 1966–2005 Embase 1980–2005 Cochrane 1800–2005 Cinahl 1982–2005
TXDF1	In patients with ACKD, what factors (including patient factors) determine the dose and frequency of ESA required to correct anaemia?	Systematic reviews, RCTs and comparative studies	Medline 1966–2005 Embase 1980–2005 Cochrane 1800–2005 Cinahl 1982–2005
TXDF2	In patients with ACKD, what factors determine the dose and frequency of ESA required to keep the haemoglobin level within the maintenance range?	Systematic reviews, RCTs and comparative studies	Medline 1966–2005 Embase 1980–2005 Cochrane 1800–2005 Cinahl 1982–2005
ESAD1	In patients with ACKD, what factors determine the provision of ESAs?	All study types	Medline 1966–2005 Embase 1980–2005 Cochrane 1800–2005 Cinahl 1982–2005
ESAD2	In patients with ACKD, what factors determine the route of administration of ESAs?	Systematic reviews, RCTs and comparative studies	Medline 1966–2005 Embase 1980–2005 Cochrane 1800–2005 Cinahl 1982–2005
NURS1	Is the effectiveness of anaemia management in chronic kidney disease improved by the involvement of anaemia nurse specialists/ coordinators?	All study types including qualitative	Medline 1966–2005 Embase 1980–2005 Cochrane 1800–2005 Cinahl 1982–2005
MON1	In patients with ACKD treated with ESAs, how frequently should iron status be checked?	All study types	Medline 1966–2005 Embase 1980–2005 Cochrane 1800–2005 Cinahl 1982–2005
MON2	In patients with ACKD treated with ESAs, how frequently should haemoglobin levels be checked a) during Hb correction and b) during Hb maintenance?	All study types	Medline 1966–2005 Embase 1980–2005 Cochrane 1800–2005 Cinahl 1982–2005
ESAR1	When should resistance to ESAs be suspected and what conditions lead to ESA resistance?	All study types	Medline 1966–2005 Embase 1980–2005 Cochrane 1800–2005 Cinahl 1982–2005
ESAR2	How should ESA resistance be managed?	All study types	Medline 1966–2005 Embase 1980–2005 Cochrane 1800–2005 Cinahl 1982–2005

NOTE: The final cut-off date for all searches was 28 September 2005.

Appendix B: Scope

Guideline title

Anaemia management in people with chronic kidney disease (CKD)

▷ Short title

Anaemia in chronic kidney disease

Background

The National Institute for Clinical Excellence ('NICE' or 'the Institute') has commissioned the National Collaborating Centre for Chronic Conditions to develop a clinical guideline on the management of anaemia in chronic kidney disease (CKD) for use in the NHS in England and Wales. This follows referral of the topic by the Department of Health and Welsh Assembly Government (see below). The guideline will provide recommendations for good practice that are based on the best available evidence of clinical and cost effectiveness.

The Institute's clinical guidelines will support the implementation of National Service Frameworks (NSFs) in those aspects of care where a Framework has been published. The statements in each NSF reflect the evidence that was used at the time the Framework was prepared. The clinical guidelines and technology appraisals published by the Institute after an NSF has been issued will have the effect of updating the Framework. The NSF for Renal Services (2004) is of particular relevance to this guideline.

Clinical need for the guideline

The NSF for Renal Services (2004) defines chronic kidney disease (CKD) as kidney (renal) disease that is irreversible and progressive. Established renal failure (also called end stage renal failure) is CKD that has progressed so far that renal replacement therapy (regular dialysis treatment or kidney transplantation) is needed to maintain life.

Established renal failure is an irreversible, long-term condition. A small number of people with established renal failure may choose conservative management only. Conventionally the total number of people receiving renal replacement therapy has been taken as a proxy measure for the prevalence of established renal failure. The NSF for Renal Services estimates that more than 27,000 people received renal replacement therapy in England in 2001. Approximately one-half of these had a functioning transplant and the remainder were on dialysis. It is predicted that numbers will rise to around 45,000 over the next 10 years. However, the most recent Renal Registry Report (2003) states that 32,500 patients received renal replacement therapy with 46% having a renal transplant.

The UK Renal Registry Report (2003) highlights that 43% of patients newly receiving dialysis had a haemoglobin level of <10 g/dl in 2002. This is despite the fact that patients receiving dialysis treatment during 2002 had haemoglobin concentrations that continued to improve.

The Registry demonstrated that 82% of haemodialysis patients and 88% of peritoneal dialysis patients had a haemoglobin concentration >10 g/dl.

The clinical need for the guideline is supported by the wide variation in practice and lack of agreement on the optimal management of renal anaemia. The UK Renal Registry Report (2003) draws attention to the fact that it was not possible to provide accurate information about erythropoietin because of variations in the recording of erythropoietin data and also the provision of erythropoietin from primary care in some parts of the UK. An evidence-based guideline should improve the standards of care across renal units and aid appropriate commissioning of cost-effective treatments.

The guideline

The guideline development process is described in detail in two publications which are available from the NICE website (see further information below). *Guideline development process – an overview for stakeholders, the public and the NHS* describes how organisations can become involved in the development of a guideline. The *Guideline development methods – information for national collaborating centres and guideline developers* provides advice on the technical aspects of guideline development.

This document is the scope. It defines exactly what this guideline will (and will not) examine, and what the guideline developers will consider. The scope is based on the referral from the Department of Health and Welsh Assembly Government (see below).

The areas that will be addressed by the guideline are described in the following sections.

Population

▷ Groups that will be covered

(a) The guideline will offer best practice advice on the care of people who have a clinical diagnosis of anaemia associated with CKD.

(b) The guideline will encompass the care of people with predialysis CKD, people with established renal failure receiving renal replacement therapy, people with established renal failure receiving conservative management, and people after renal transplant surgery.

(c) The guideline will cover children (aged <16 years).

▷ Groups that will not be covered

Where CKD is not the principal cause of the anaemia it will be excluded, for example:

- anaemia caused by haematological disease
- anaemia caused by acute and chronic inflammatory disease states
- anaemia caused by malignancy
- anaemia caused by acquired immunodeficiency syndrome
- anaemia caused by acute renal failure.

Healthcare setting

The guideline will cover the care provided by healthcare professionals in direct contact with patients with anaemia associated with CKD and make decisions about their care. This will include healthcare professionals in primary, secondary and tertiary NHS care settings.

Clinical management

The guideline will include recommendations in the following areas.

(a) Detection and diagnosis of anaemia in people with CKD:
- exclusion of other causes of anaemia
- diagnostic evaluation of anaemia in CKD
- assessment of anaemia.

(b) Criteria for the threshold levels of haemoglobin concentration for initiating the treatment of anaemia.

(c) Factors which have an impact on anaemia in renal disease and their management including:
- nutritional status including haematinics
- dialysis adequacy (peritoneal and haemodialysis)
- hyperparathyroidism
- assessment and optimisation of erythropoiesis to include iron stores, iron supplements and erythropoiesis stimulating agents
- monitoring of treatment of anaemia associated with people with CKD.

Guideline recommendations will normally fall within licensed indications; exceptionally, and only where clearly supported by evidence, use outside a licensed indication may be recommended. The guideline will assume that prescribers will use the Summary of product characteristics to inform their decisions for individual patients.

Status

▷ Scope

This is the final version of the scope.

▷ Guideline

The development of the guideline recommendations will begin in October 2004.

Further information

Information on the guideline development process is provided in:
- *Guideline development process – an overview for stakeholders, the public and the NHS*
- *Guideline development methods – information for national collaborating centres and guideline developers*

These booklets are available as PDF files from the NICE website (**www.nice.org.uk**). Information on the progress of the guideline will also be available from the website.

Referral from the Department of Health and Welsh Assembly Government

The Department of Health and Welsh Assembly Government asked the Institute:

'To develop a guideline for the NHS in England and Wales for the management of anaemia in people with poor renal function, including chronic kidney disease and established renal failure, based on evidence of clinical and cost effectiveness of interventions available for treating anaemia in such people. The interventions should be all those factors that have an impact on anaemia including nutritional status, dialysis effectiveness, iron stores and the use of recombinant human erythropoietin. The purpose of the guideline will be to take renal staff and patients through the most cost-effective set of investigations and procedures which will optimise haemoglobin and if possible keep it above the accepted international standard, for example European and K-DOQI of 11 g/dl.'

Appendix C: Health economic model: target haemoglobin in haemodialysis patients

Background

The treatment of anaemia in CKD helps increase the health-related quality of life of patients. However, the optimal haemoglobin target continues to be debated. While there is an economic evaluation on the cost effectiveness of different targets based on US data, the lack of cost-effectiveness data in the UK warranted further investigation.

Aim

The aim of the model is to compare three alternative haemoglobin (Hb) targets in the anaemia management of haemodialysis patients over a 2-year period. The haemoglobin targets evaluated were: <11 g/dl, 11–12 g/dl and >12 g/dl. The cost per quality-adjusted life year gained was calculated.

Methods

A cost-effectiveness model was constructed from the perspective of the NHS. The effectiveness outcome measure used was quality-adjusted life years (QALYs) and the incremental cost per QALY was calculated. Point estimates are derived from probabilistic results.

Incremental cost per QALY = $(C_1 - C_2) / (Q_1 - Q_2)$

Where:

C_1 = Estimated cost of anaemia treatment to reach Hb target

C_2 = Estimated cost of anaemia treatment to reach higher Hb target

Q_1 = Estimated quality-adjusted life years from Hb target

Q_2 = Estimated quality-adjusted life years from higher Hb target

The data sources of the costs and benefits are described in further detail in Tables C.1–C.4. All costs and benefits were discounted at an annual rate of 3.5% in accordance with current NICE recommendations in their *Guideline development methods* 2005. Costs and benefits were accrued monthly over the 2-year period. A 1-month cycle was chosen as blood tests are routinely taken monthly in haemodialysis patients. A 2-year time horizon was chosen as it was considered a clinically relevant time period of treatment considering transplantation rates and survival on dialysis. The 11–12 g/dl haemoglobin target was selected based on the GDG's interpretation of the clinical data. This alternative was compared with below 11 g/dl and above 12 g/dl to assess the cost effectiveness of these alternative strategies. All costs are in pound sterling with base-year 2005. One-way sensitivity analysis and a cost-effectiveness acceptability curve were constructed to assess the impact of uncertainty on the incremental cost-effectiveness ratio (ICER). Threshold analyses were performed to investigate the value of the utility of Hb target 11–12 g/dl for which the ICER becomes £30,000.

Data sources and assumptions

Tables C.1–C.4 list the baseline cost and effectiveness outcomes along with the sources of data. Assumptions and methods of calculating estimates are described in further detail below.

Table C.1 Dose of ESA for each Hb target range				
Model target Hb (g/dl)	Hb target in source study (g/dl)	Type of ESA	IU/wk	Source
<11	10 + 1	Epoetin-alfa	10,671 (SD 7,236, n=18)	293
11–12	>11.0	Epoetin-alfa/beta s.c. and i.v.	10,831 (n=189)*	294
>12	13.5–16.0	Epoetin-alfa s.c.	236 (U/kg/wk) (SD 148, n=157)	295
			15,340** (SD 148.3, n=157)	(Estimate)

* No standard deviation given in study. Assumed same %SD of IU/wk as <11. (67.8%, estimated SD 7,344).
** Assuming 65 + 10 kg average weight.

Mean epoetin values in Table C.1 were derived from RCT data where possible and selected based on the target haemoglobins in the studies being the closest to <11, 11–12 and >12 g/dl.

The cost of epoetin was calculated using a unit cost of £7.96 for 1,000 units of epoetin alfa and pre-filled syringe from the British national formulary (BNF) 49.

Table C.2 Calculations per month	
IU/month of ESA	Cost per month (£)
46,398.80	369.33
47,094.50	374.87
66,700.18	530.93

Table C.3 All-cause mortality[46]			
Hb (g/dl)	Deaths/1,000 treatment-yr (adjusted)*	RR (adjusted) per month cycle: (mortality rate, standard error)	Deaths/1,000 treatment-yr (unadjusted)
< 11	249	1.25 (.021, .0045)	259
11–12	199	1 (.016, .0040)	199
>12	197	0.99 (.016, .0040)	192

*Calculated using unadjusted rate and RR.

Model target Hb (g/dl)	Hb target in source study (g/dl)	Value	Measurement technique	n	Source
< 11	9.5–11.0 (10.2 + 1.0)	0.51	Time trade off	34	142
11–12	-	0.545	–		(estimate)*
>12	11.5–13.0 (11.7 + 1.4)	0.58	Time trade off	33	142

Table C.4 Utility score

* Estimated the utility score of the Hb target 11–12 g/dl as the midpoint between the values for target Hb<11 and Hb>12. (.545).
Note: no standard deviation given in study. Standard error of .02 (~10%SD) for each utility value.

Explanation of assumptions and data used

▷   Costs

Only costs specific to anaemia treatment rather than haemodialysis care and those that are different between the treatment strategies were included.

Hb target <11 g/dl

The monthly cost of reaching the Hb target was derived from the mean dose of ESA per week used in a randomised open-label trial comparing target Hb of 10 + 1 g/dl and 14 + 1 g/dl in 35 dialysis patients[293] and the unit cost of epoetin alfa in a pre-filled syringe. The total cost of care per patient was considered stable for the 2-year period.

Hb target 11–12 g/dl

The monthly cost of Hb target 11–12 g/dl was derived from the mean epoetin dose from the Results of the European Survey on Anaemia Management in 2003 (ESAM)[294] based on 189 haemodialysis, haemofiltration and haemofiltration patients in the UK and the unit cost of epoetin alfa in a pre-filled syringe.

Hb target >12 g/dl

The monthly cost of Hb target >12 g/dl was derived from the mean U/kg/week of epoetin from a randomised controlled trial of 157 haemodialysis patients treated to a target Hb range of 13.5–16.0 g/dl and the unit cost of epoetin alfa in a pre-filled syringe. It was assumed an average patient would be 65 + 10 kg in order to calculate the mean units/week.

Other cost drivers that were assumed to be the same regardless of the Hb target range were:
● consultation time and type of health professional responsible for anaemia management
● iron strategy
● haemodialysis treatment (considered part of standard care).

▷ Quality-adjusted life years

Hb target <11 g/dl, Hb target >12 g/dl

The quality of life in Hb target <11 g/dl and Hb target >12 g/dl were derived from a randomised study comparing placebo, 9.5–11.0 g/dl and 11.5–13.0 g/dl achieved Hb ranges in 118 haemodialysis. The results from the time trade off technique were used as the QALY weight in the estimation of QALYs. Although these were achieved Hb ranges, it was assumed that a target of >12 g/dl or <11 g/dl would have achieved haemoglobin levels similar to these ranges. Total QALY gain in each month cycle was added with a 3.5% annual discount rate.

Hb target 11–12 g/dl

The quality of life in target Hb 11–12 g/dl was estimated as the midpoint between the values for target Hb <11 and Hb >12. (.545) This method of estimation was chosen on the following reasoning from the clinical evidence:

In quality of life studies > 6 months in duration there is statistically significant quality of life improvement in certain dimensions such as physical functioning.

There is significant improvement between 9.0–12.0 and 13.5–16.0 g/dl,[295] 10 and 14 g/dl[207] and 10.2 and 12.5 g/dl.[49] There is improvement (but not significant) between 9.5–11.0 and 11.5–13.0.[142] This suggests that the quality of life between 11 and 12 is probably not the same as >12, and probably is slightly less than it is in Hb >12 and more than <11, suggesting a linear estimation is reasonable.

Additional assumptions

- There is no increased risk of access failure or hypertension with higher haemoglobin targets.
- Concordance.
- Rate of transplantation is equivalent in each treatment strategy.
- Dialysis adequacy is equivalent in each treatment strategy.
- Mean epoetin doses remain representative of costs over a 2-year period.
- There is no difference in hospitalisation rates with different haemoglobin targets.

Observational studies suggest a difference in the number of hospitalisations and reduction in duration of stays,[46,49] however, it is very possible these values were not adjusted sufficiently for confounders. Two RCTs[207,295] and the meta-analysis[202] indicate there is no significant difference in rate and days of hospitalisation. Therefore, the rate of hospitalisation was not used in the model to differentiate between Hb targets.

Mortality rates

The mortality rates used in the model were derived from the adjusted relative risk of death and all-cause mortality rates in patients in an observational study of 66,761 patients.[46] The GDG felt the evidence on mortality in the meta-analysis[202] may be more biased by the weight given to one study on patients with cardiovascular disease[207] than the observational study.

Results

Table C.5 Probabilistic model results: 2-year time horizon		
Hb range (g/dl)	Cost (£)	QALYs
<11	7,202	0.79
11–12	7,750	0.90
>12	10,993	0.97

Table C.6 Probabilistic incremental results of baseline values			
Hb range (g/dl)	Incremental cost (£)	Incremental QALYs	ICER (£ per QALY)
11–12 vs <11	548	0.11	4,985
>12 vs 11–12	3,242	0.07	47,458

Note: differences due to rounding.

Sensitivity analysis

The estimates used in the model are subject to uncertainty. Therefore, a one-way sensitivity analysis was carried out to assess the impact of key variables used in the model. A one-way sensitivity analysis varies one parameter while maintaining the other parameters at baseline values. The variables included reflect the mortality rates, costs, utilities and hospitalisation rates used in the deterministic model. Results for the upper and lower estimates are given in Tables C.7 and C.8.

Table C.7 One-way sensitivity analysis				
Variable	Baseline value	Range evaluated	Hb comparison	ICER range estimate (dominant strategy)
RR death Hb <11	1.25	1.20 1.30	11–12 vs <11	4,369 4,999
RR death Hb >12	0.99	0.92 1.07	>12 vs 11–12	46,906 69,224
Cost per month cycle Hb <11 (£)	369.33	118.89 619.78	11–12 vs <11	55,808 Hb11–12
Cost per month cycle Hb 11–12 (£)	374.87	120.67 629.07	11–12 vs <11	Hb11–12 59,007
			>12 vs 11–12	143,557 Hb>12
Cost per month cycle Hb >12 (£)	530.93	525.80 536.07	>12 vs 11–12	53,026 56,617

continued

143

Table C.7 One-way sensitivity analysis – *continued*

Variable	Baseline value	Range evaluated	Hb comparison	ICER range estimate (dominant strategy)
Utility Hb <11	0.51	0.46 0.56	11–12 vs <11	2,589 26,632
Utility Hb 11–12	0.55	0.49 0.60	11–12 vs <11	61,140 2,454
			>12 vs 11–12	21,856 Hb11–12
Utility Hb>12	0.58	0.52 0.64	>12 vs 11–12	Hb 11–12 21,018

Table C.8 Sensitivity analysis of hospitalisation risks and costs

	Baseline Estimates (No difference)	Observational Study Estimates	Cost of hospitalisation (£)
RR of hospitalisation Hb <11	1.0	1.21	2,190
RR of hospitalisation Hb 11–12	1.0	1.0	
RR of hospitalisation Hb >12	1.0	0.78	
ICER Hb11–12 vs Hb<11	4,719	1,444	
ICER Hb>12 vs Hb11–12	54,822	41,481	
ICER Hb11–12 vs Hb<11		3,719	863 (lower estimate)
ICER Hb>12 vs Hb11–12		46,750	
ICER Hb11–12 vs Hb<11		84	2,983 (upper estimate)
ICER Hb>12 vs Hb11–12		38,333	

The extent of uncertainty in the probabilistic model is displayed in Figure C.1.

Figure C.2 summarises into probabilities the uncertainty that an alternative is cost effective for a range of willingness-to-pay thresholds.

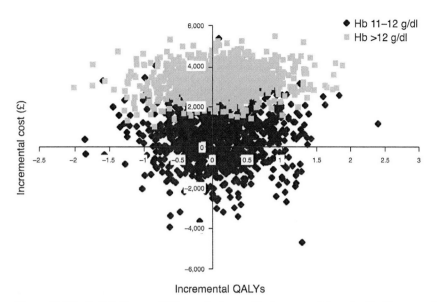

Figure C.1 Probabilistic sensitivity analysis results: incremental cost-effectiveness plane

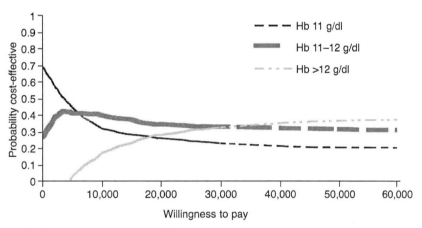

Figure C.2 Cost-effectiveness acceptability curve (£)

Discussion

Point estimates suggest Hb target 11–12 g/dl is the optimal strategy with a £20,000–30,000 threshold. Uncertainty was assessed in the deterministic results in a one-way and two-way sensitivity analyses (Tables C.7 and C.8). At the upper estimate of the monthly cost of Hb 11–12 (£629.07), target Hb 11–12 is dominated by Hb >12: the total costs in Hb 11–12 are higher than Hb >12 but results in less QALYs. While the upper estimate is a plausible estimate of Hb 11–12, it would mean the unlikely situation, in the absence of hospitalisation costs saved, where the monthly cost to reach Hb >12 is less than the monthly cost to reach Hb 11–12 (£530.93).

At the lower estimate of Hb 11–12 utility, the Hb 11–12 vs Hb<11 ICER increased to £61,140 and the Hb >12 vs Hb 11–12 ICER increased to £21,856. The lower estimate of Hb 11–12 (0.49) is less than the baseline estimate of Hb <11 (0.51), contrary to clinical evidence. Rather than make an assumption about the utility of Hb target 11–12 g/dl per month, if we allow the utility to vary, the value at which the ICER of 11–12 g/dl vs <11 g/dl target is £30,000 is 0.50. This would mean the utility of target Hb 11–12 g/dl would have to be less than the utility of target Hb <11 g/dl (0.51) in order for the target Hb 11–12 g/dl not to be cost effective as defined by an ICER of £30,000 or less.

At the higher estimate of Hb 11–12 utility, Hb 11–12 vs Hb <11 ICER decreased to £2,454 and the Hb 11–12 dominates Hb >12 (in this case Hb 11–12 costs less with more QALYs gained). This is reasonable as the same costs and more QALYs gained in Hb 11–12 will result in more favourable ICERs.

At the lower estimate of the utility of Hb >12, the Hb 11–12 strategy dominates Hb >12 (in this case Hb 12 costs more with less QALYs gained), however, at the upper estimate, the Hb >12 vs Hb 11–12 ICER decreased to £21,018.

Similarly, if we allow the utility of target Hb 11–12 g/dl to vary, the value at which the ICER of >12 g/dl vs 11–12 g/dl is £30,000 is 0.52. This would mean the utility of target Hb 11–12 g/dl would be much closer to the Hb <11 g/dl (0.51) rather than the utility of target Hb >12 g/dl (0.58) in order for the target Hb >12 g/dl to be cost effective as defined by an ICER of £30,000 or less.

If the baseline rates of hospitalisations are changed from the assumption that rates are equivalent in each Hb target to the adjusted rates in the observational study,[46] hospitalisation requires a cost. The national average unit cost of acute renal failure (£2,190) with upper (£2,983) and lower (£863) ranges of this unit cost was used in the sensitivity analysis of hospitalisation rates. ICERS with the lower and upper range of this unit cost were calculated to assess if there was an effect of the size of the cost of hospitalisation on the results. The Hb 11–12 vs Hb <11 ICER decreased from 4,719 to 1,444 (hospitalisation cost £2,190), 3,719 (hospitalisation cost £863) and 84 (hospitalisation cost £2,983) further in favour of Hb 11–12. The ICER Hb >12 vs Hb 11–12 also decreased 54,822 to 41,481 (£2,190), 46,750 (£863), 38,333 (£2,983). However these remain above a £30,000 cost-effectiveness threshold.

In probabilistic analysis, each parameter is assigned a distribution such as beta, normal, gamma and so on, and random values from these distributions are used to derive cost-effectiveness results. The extent of uncertainty in the model is displayed in Figure C.1. The scatter of the estimates indicates a high degree of uncertainty over the four quadrants. The cost-effectiveness acceptability curve (CEAC) (Figure C.2) summarises the uncertainty of the results. For every value on the x-axis third-party payers are willing to pay, the probability the alternative is cost effective is indicated on the y-axis. Between £20,000 to £30,000 willingness-to-pay threshold, the Hb target 11–12 g/dl has the highest probability of cost effectiveness (0.378 to 0.365), suggesting Hb 11–12 g/dl is the best choice of the three alternatives. Even though the strategy has the highest probability of cost effectiveness, there still is a large amount of uncertainty that could be improved with better data, especially compared with >12 g/dl.

The benefits in this model were assessed for a 2-year period only. This means life-time costs and benefits of treatments were not analysed. Also, the results were based on haemodialysis patients, rather than all CKD patients. If possible, randomised studies with target haemoglobin ranges corresponding to <11, 11–12 and >12 g/dl were selected. However, individuals will clinically respond differently to epoetin and there may be different distributions of achieved haemoglobin across the haemodialysis population with particular haemoglobin targets. The number of people who achieved the target was not taken into account in the selection of the data sources because of the limited reporting in the literature. The mean epoetin value for the <11 g/dl was based on an appropriate study target range, but there was a small number of patients.[293] The 11–12 g/dl epoetin value was based on a European survey where guidelines suggest an 11–12 g/dl target. The target haemoglobin range in the[295] study was 1.5 g/dl higher than 12, which may have increased the amount of epoetin needed to reach higher than 12 while the quality of life data was from a lower haemoglobin (11.5–13.0 g/dl). The mean epoetin data sources combined three haemodialysis populations from the USA, UK and Scandinavia potentially reducing the generalisability to the UK population. Therefore this is a preliminary analysis until further economic and clinical outcomes are measured.

The results are similar to the US study[208] that found dosing epoetin to Hb >12.0 g/dl had unfavourable cost-effectiveness ratios. However, comparative target Hb ranges, costs included, such as cost of hospitalisation, haemodialysis care, renal transplantation, epoetin dosages and time horizon (life-time of patient) were different between the studies which may make comparing direct results inappropriate. Of note, the incremental cost per QALY gained in the 12.0–12.5 vs 11.0–12.0 g/dl comparison was approximately 11 times greater than the 11.0–12.0 vs 9.5–10.5 g/dl in the US study, whereas in this UK analysis the >12 vs 11–12 is approximately 9.5 times greater than the 11–12 vs <11 g/dl incremental cost per QALY gained.

Conclusion

The results suggest treating anaemia with a target Hb 11–12 g/dl is cost effective in haemodialysis patients based on a £30,000 threshold. However, there is uncertainty in the results of the model from lack of certainty in the input parameters. Nevertheless, the results are relatively robust based on one-way sensitivity analyses and threshold analyses. This analysis is a simplified model of the costs and benefits of treating anaemia in the haemodialysis population and a variety of assumptions have been used in the baseline analysis. Therefore, the results should be interpreted correspondingly.

Appendix D: Health economic calculation: route of administration of ESAs

Background

▷ Aim

To perform a cost-minimisation analysis based on equivalent effectiveness between intravenous (i.v.) and subcutaneous (s.c.) epoetin. ESAs are made available to NHS trusts through a system of tendering for local supply contracts. Costs therefore vary between locations and over time, and this should be borne in mind in applying the findings of this analysis.

▷ Methods

A cost-minimisation model was constructed from the perspective of the NHS. Cost analysis included epoetin, iron, administration and potential wastage. A meta-analysis of randomised controlled trials comparing i.v. and s.c. doses required to maintain target haematocrit or haemoglobin levels was performed to derive the average dose difference of i.v. and s.c. Other resource use was estimated by expert opinion and the trials used in the meta-analysis.

Incremental cost = $(C_1 - C_2)$

Where:

C_1 = Estimated cost of i.v. epoetin therapy
C_2 = Estimated cost of s.c. epoetin therapy

Data sources

▷ Costs

Subcutaneous epoetin

Table D.1 Unit cost of subcutaneous epoetin beta[BNF49]		
Subcutaneous epoetin beta	Units	Price (£)
	10,000	77.93
	20,000	155.87
	60,000	467.61

The average cost per unit of s.c. epoetin used in cost calculations was £0.007793.

▷ Other costs

Iron

Only one of the three studies included in the meta-analysis reported the average total amounts of iron administered per patient during all phases.[172] No significant differences in average total amount of parenteral iron dextran were found between the i.v. and s.c. groups within the study (1,683 + 1,280 vs 1,765 + 1,342, p=0.65). Expert opinion indicated there would be an equivalent iron strategy in clinical practice regardless of the route of administration of epoetin. Therefore the cost difference of iron with i.v. or s.c. epoetin was assumed to be negligible.

Administration

Expert opinion suggested the same health professional would administer i.v. or s.c. epoetin, the healthcare setting would not need to be changed and wastage would be similar with either i.v. or s.c. administration. Two studies reported there was no significant difference in mean dialysis time.[132,175] Therefore the cost difference of administration with i.v. or s.c. epoetin was assumed to be negligible.

Dose differences

Three randomised controlled trials[132,172,175] were used to derive the mean difference and 95% confidence interval of i.v. and s.c. dose in a fixed meta-analysis. Only studies receiving a 1++ or 1+ in the NICE levels of evidence hierarchy in the clinical effectiveness review and with n >7 were included. The average dose difference of patients treated with s.c. vs i.v. epoetin was 41.61 IU/kg/wk (95% CI 22.55 − 60.66) (p=0.000). Drug cost differences were calculated using the median unit cost in the base-case and the 95% confidence interval to calculate the range of cost savings per week and per year.

Results

Based on a unit cost of £0.007793 per unit of epoetin and a 65 + 10 kg patient, the average cost savings per patient with s.c. epoetin vs i.v. epoetin was £21.08 + £13.93 per week. The average yearly cost savings with s.c. epoetin was £1,100 + £727 per patient.

Discussion

There are potential drug cost savings when using s.c. epoetin instead of i.v. epoetin to maintain target haematocrit or haemoglobin levels. These savings occur in supervised healthcare settings; however, self-administration in the patient's home with s.c. epoetin is an alternative anaemia management strategy. Further evidence including delivery costs, gaining health professional time and treatment-related outcomes during self-management would be needed to assess different service provision strategies.

Darbepoetin is an alternative drug used in the management of anaemia in chronic kidney disease. Darbepoetin can be used by both the s.c. and i.v. routes of administration. However, because of the lack of data it was not included. When further data is available, this analysis could include the cost effectiveness of darbepoetin s.c. vs i.v. and darbepoetin vs epoetin.

A potential consideration of s.c. vs i.v. administration of epoetin that may vary on an individual level is patient preference due to potential pain at the injection site. One of the included randomised trials measured the discomfort during treatment.[172] Of 96 patients who had received both routes of administration, 74% preferred i.v. and 26% had no preference or preferred s.c. Eight of 24 (33%) at the start of treatment with s.c. epoetin had pain at the injection site, however, only one of these patients had pain at the end of study (4 months).[175] 31% of patients reported pain during placebo subcutaneous injection during the run-in period and only 18% reported pain during epoetin subcutaneous injection.[132]

Conclusion

The subcutaneous route of administration of epoetin vs intravenous route results in cost savings of approximately £1,100 + £727 per patient per year.

Appendix E: Glossary

Abbreviations

ACKD	Anaemia of chronic kidney disease
bd	Twice daily
CAPD	Continuous ambulatory peritoneal dialysis
CCr	Creatinine clearance
CI	Confidence interval
CKD	Chronic kidney disease
DM	Diabetes mellitus
DS	Diagnostic study
eGFR	Estimated glomerular filtration rate
EPO	Erythropoietin
ESA	Erythropoiesis stimulating agent
FID	Functional iron deficiency
GI	Gastrointestinal
GFR	Glomerular filtration rate
GPP	Good practice point
Hb	Haemoglobin
Hct	Haematocrit
HD	Haemodialysis
HR	Hazard ratio
HRC	Hypochromic red cells
IP	Intraperitoneal
i.v.	Intravenously
LVH	Left ventricular hypertrophy
MCV	Mean corpuscular volume
MI	Myocardial infarction
NHS	National Health Service
NICE	National Institute for Health and Clinical Excellence
NSF	National service framework
PD	Peritoneal dialysis
PRCA	Pure red cell aplasia
PTX	Parathyroidectomy
RCT	Randomised controlled trial
RES	Reticuloendothelial system
ROC	Receiver-operator curve
RR	Relative risk

s.c.	Subcutaneous
s.c.r	Serum creatinine
tds	Three times daily
TSAT	Transferrin saturation
WMD	Weighted mean difference
ZPP	(Erythrocyte) zinc protoporphyrin

Guide to assessment scales

Health related quality of life (HRQL)	A combination of a person's physical, mental and social well-being; not merely the absence of disease.
Renal Quality of Life Profile	A quality of life scale developed and validated specifically for people with renal disease.
Short Form 36 (SF-36)	The SF-36 assesses functioning and well-being in chronic disease. Thirty-six items in eight domains are included, which cover functional status, well-being, and overall evaluation of health.
Sickness Impact Profile (SIP)	SIP is a general quality of life scale. It consists of 136 items, which measure 12 distinct domains of quality of life. Participants identify those statements, which describe their experience. Higher scores represent greater dysfunction.
Visual Analogue Scale (VAS)	A non-graduated 100 mm vertical line ranging from '0=no pain' to '100=pain as bad as could be'. Patients indicate pain sensation by scoring on the vertical line with a horizontal dash.
Verbal Descriptive Scale (VDS)	Divided into the following six categories: no pain, hardly any pain, mild pain, moderate pain, severe pain, unbearable pain. Patients tick the appropriate category on a questionnaire

Stages of chronic kidney disease

Stage	GFR (ml/min/1.73m^2)	Description
1	>90	Normal or increased GFR, with other evidence of kidney damage
2	60–89	Slight decrease in GFR, with other evidence of kidney damage
3	30–59	Moderate decrease in GFR, with or without other evidence of kidney damage
4	15–29	Severe decrease in GFR, with or without other evidence of kidney damage
5	<15	Established renal failure

Definition of terms

Absolute iron deficiency	Depletion in iron body stores.
Adverse events	A harmful, and usually relatively rare, event arising from treatment.
Algorithm (in guidelines)	A flow chart of the clinical decision pathway described in the guideline.
Allocation concealment	The process used to prevent advance knowledge of group assignment in an RCT, and potential bias that may result.
Anaemia coordinator	A healthcare professional who is a central point of contact for patients with ACKD – see recommendation R28 in section 6.5.3 for details.
Audit	See 'clinical audit'.
Before and after study	See 'observational study'.
Bias	The effect that the results of a study are not an accurate reflection of any trends in the wider population. This may result from flaws in the design of a study or in the analysis of results.
Blinding (masking)	A feature of study design to keep the participants, researchers and outcome assessors unaware of the interventions that have been allocated.
Carer (caregiver)	Someone other than a health professional who is involved in caring for a person with a medical condition, such as a relative or spouse.
Case-control study	Comparative observational study in which the investigator selects individuals who have experienced an event (for example, developed a disease) and others who have not (controls), and then collects data to determine previous exposure to a possible cause.
Class of recommendation	All recommendations are assigned a class (A, B, C, D, A(DS), B(DS), C(DS), or D(GPP)) according to the level of evidence the recommendation is based on (see 'level of evidence').
Clinical audit	A quality improvement process that seeks to improve patient care and outcomes through systematic review of care against explicit criteria and the implementation of change.
Clinician	In this guideline, the term clinician means any healthcare professional.
Cochrane review	A systematic review of the evidence from randomised controlled trials relating to a particular health problem or healthcare intervention, produced by the Cochrane Collaboration. Available electronically as part of the Cochrane Library.
Cohort study	A retrospective or prospective follow-up study. Groups of individuals to be followed up are defined on the basis of presence or absence of exposure to a suspected risk factor or intervention. A cohort study can be comparative, in which case two or more groups are selected on the basis of differences in their exposure to the agent of interest.
Concordance	Concordance is a concept reflecting agreement between clinicians and patient on the best course of managing a disease, and adherence to that course until alternatives are agreed on and adopted.
Confidence interval (CI)	A range of values which contains the true value for the population with a stated 'confidence' (conventionally 95%). The interval is calculated from sample data, and generally straddles the sample estimate. The 95% confidence value means that if the study, and the method used to calculate the interval, is repeated many times, then 95% of the calculated intervals will actually contain the true value for the whole population.
Cost-effectiveness analysis	An economic study design in which consequences of different interventions are measured using a single outcome, usually in natural units (for example, life years gained, deaths avoided, heart attacks avoided, cases detected). Alternative interventions are then compared in terms of cost per unit of effectiveness.
Cost-effectiveness model	An explicit mathematical framework, which is used to represent clinical decision problems and incorporate evidence from a variety of sources in order to estimate the costs and health outcomes.

Cost-utility analysis	A form of cost-effectiveness analysis in which the units of effectiveness are quality-adjusted life years (QALYs).
Cycling	See 'haemoglobin cycling'.
Diagnostic study	Any research study aimed at evaluating the utility of a diagnostic procedure.
Erythropoiesis	Red blood cell production.
Evidence-based healthcare	The process of systematically finding, appraising, and using research findings as the basis for clinical decisions.
Follow up	An attempt to measure the outcomes of an intervention after the intervention has ended.
Functional iron deficiency	Inadequate iron mobilisation, which is incapable of meeting demands of erythropoiesis.
Generalisability	The degree to which the results of a study or systematic review can be extrapolated to other circumstances, particularly routine healthcare situations in the NHS in England and Wales.
Gold standard	See 'reference standard'.
Good Practice Point	Recommended good practice based on the clinical experience of the Guideline Development Group.
Grade of recommendation	See 'class of recommendation'.
Guideline development group (GDG)	An independent group set up on behalf of NICE to develop a guideline. They include healthcare professionals and patient and carer representatives.
Haematocrit	Relative volume of blood occupied by red blood cells.
Haemoglobin cycling	Fluctuation of haemoglobin levels which may vary from patient to patient.
Hazard ratio (HR)	A statistic to describe the relative risk of complications due to treatment, based on a comparison of event rates.
Heterogeneity	In systematic reviews, heterogeneity refers to variability or differences between studies in estimates of effect.
Homogeneity	In a systematic review, homogeneity means there are no or minor variations in the results between individual studies included in a systematic review.
Inclusion criteria	Explicit criteria used to decide which studies should be considered as potential sources of evidence.
Incremental cost	The cost of one alternative less the cost of another.
Incremental cost-effectiveness ratio (ICER)	The ratio of the difference in costs between two alternatives to the difference in effectiveness between the same two alternatives.
Intention-to-treat analysis (ITT analysis)	An analysis of the results of a clinical study in which the data are analysed for all study participants as if they had remained in the group to which they were randomised, regardless of whether or not they remained in the study until the end, crossed over to another treatment or received an alternative intervention.
Level of evidence	A code (eg 1++, 1+,2++) linked to an individual study, indicating where it fits into the NICE hierarchy of evidence and how well it has adhered to recognised research principles.
Meta-analysis	A statistical technique for combining (pooling) the results of a number of studies that address the same question and report on the same outcomes to produce a summary result.
Methodological limitations	Features of the design or reporting of a clinical study, which are known to be associated with risk of bias or lack of validity. Where a study is reported in this guideline as having significant methodological limitations, a recommendation has not been directly derived from it.
Multivariate model	A statistical model for analysis of the relationship between two or more predictor (independent) variables and the outcome (dependent) variable.

National Collaborating Centre for Chronic Conditions (NCC-CC)	A partnership of the Clinical Effectiveness Forum for Allied Health Professions, the NHS Confederation, the NICE Patient and Public Involvement Programme, the Royal College of General Practitioners, the Royal College of Nursing, the Royal College of Physicians of London, the Royal College of Physicians' Patient Involvement Unit, the Royal College of Surgeons of England, and the Royal Pharmaceutical Society of Great Britain. Set up in 2001 to undertake commissions from NICE to develop clinical guidelines for the NHS.
National Health Service (NHS)	This guideline is written for the NHS in England and Wales.
National Institute for Health and Clinical Excellence (NICE)	NICE is the independent organisation responsible for providing national guidance on the promotion of good health and the prevention and treatment of ill health.
Negative predictive value	The proportion of people with a negative test result who do not have the disease.
Observational study	Retrospective or prospective study in which the investigator observes the natural course of events with or without control groups, for example cohort studies and case-control studies.
Odds ratio	A measure of treatment effectiveness. The odds of an event happening in the intervention group, divided by the odds of it happening in the control group. The 'odds' is the ratio of non-events to events.
Outcome	Measure of the possible results that may stem from exposure to prevention or therapeutic intervention. Outcome measures may be intermediate endpoints or they can be final endpoints.
p-values	The probability that an observed difference could have occurred by chance. A p-value of less than 0.05 is conventionally considered to be 'statistically significant'.
Placebo	An inactive and physically indistinguishable substitute for a medication or procedure, used as a comparator in controlled clinical trials.
Positive predictive value (PPV)	The proportion of people with a positive test result who actually have the disease.
Pure red cell aplasia (PRCA)	Transitory arrest of erythropoiesis.
Quality of life	Refers to the level of comfort, enjoyment, and ability to pursue daily activities.
Quality-adjusted life year (QALY)	A measure of health outcome which assigns to each period of time a weight, ranging from 0 to 1, corresponding to the health-related quality of life during that period, where a weight of 1 corresponds to optimal health, and a weight of 0 corresponds to a health state judged equivalent to death; these are then aggregated across time periods.
Randomisation	Allocation of participants in a study to two or more alternative groups using a chance procedure, such as computer-generated random numbers. This approach is used in an attempt to reduce sources of bias.
Randomised controlled trial (RCT)	A comparative study in which participants are randomly allocated to intervention and control groups and followed up to examine differences in outcomes between the groups.
Reference standard (or gold standard)	An agreed desirable standard, for example a diagnostic test or treatment, against which other interventions can be compared.
Relative risk (RR)	An estimate for the number of times more likely or less likely an event is to happen in one group of people compared with another, based on the incidence of the event in the intervention arm of a study, divided by the incidence in the control arm.
Sample size	The number of participants included in a trial or intervention group.
Sensitivity (of a test)	The proportion of people classified as positive by the gold standard, who are correctly identified by the study test.
Sensitivity analysis	A measure of the extent to which small changes in parameters and variables affect a result calculated from them. In this guideline, sensitivity analysis is used in health economic modelling.

Single blind study	A study where the investigator is aware of the treatment or intervention the participant is being given, but the participant is unaware.
Specialist	A clinician whose practice is limited to a particular branch of medicine or surgery, especially one who is certified by a higher medical educational organisation.
Specificity (of a test)	The proportion of people classified as negative by the gold standard, who are correctly identified by the study test.
Stakeholder	Any national organisation, including patient and carers' groups, healthcare professionals and commercial companies with an interest in the guideline under development.
Statistical power	In clinical trials, the probability of correctly detecting an underlying difference of a pre-specified size due to the intervention or treatment under consideration. Power is determined by the study design, and in particular, the sample size. Larger sample sizes increase the chance of small effects being correctly detected as statistically significant, though they may not be clinically significant.
Statistical significance	A result is deemed statistically significant if the probability of the result occurring by chance is less than 1 in 20 ($p<0.05$).
Systematic review	Research that summarises the evidence on a clearly formulated question according to a pre-defined protocol using systematic and explicit methods to identify, select and appraise relevant studies, and to extract, collate and report their findings. It may or may not use statistical meta-analysis.
Washout period	The stage in a crossover trial when one treatment is withdrawn before the second treatment is given.
Withdrawal	When a trial participant discontinues the assigned intervention before completion of the study.

References

1   National Institute for Clinical Excellence. *Guideline development methods. Information for national collaborating centres and guideline developers. March 2005 Update.* London: 2005.

2   World Health Organization. *Iron Deficiency Anaemia, Assessment, Prevention and Control: a guide for programme managers.* 2001.

3   Guralnik JM, Eisenstaedt RS, Ferrucci L et al. Prevalence of anemia in persons 65 years and older in the United States: evidence for a high rate of unexplained anemia. *Blood.* 2004;104(8):2263–2268.

4   Zakai NA, Katz R, Hirsch C et al. A prospective study of anemia status, hemoglobin concentration, and mortality in an elderly cohort: the Cardiovascular Health Study. *Archives of Internal Medicine.* 2005; 165(19):2214–2220.

5   Garn SM, Smith NJ, Clark DC. Lifelong differences in hemoglobin levels between blacks and whites. *Journal of the National Medical Association.* 1975;67(2):91–96.

6   Dallman PR, Barr GD, Allen CM et al. Hemoglobin concentration in white, black, and Oriental children: is there a need for separate criteria in screening for anemia? *American Journal of Clinical Nutrition.* 1978; 31(3):377–380.

7   Pan WH, Habicht JP. The non-iron-deficiency-related difference in hemoglobin concentration distribution between blacks and whites and between men and women. *American Journal of Epidemiology.* 1991;134(12):1410–1416.

8   Perry GS, Byers T, Yip R et al. Iron nutrition does not account for the hemoglobin differences between blacks and whites. *Journal of Nutrition.* 1992;122(7):1417–1424.

9   Johnson-Spear MA, Yip R. Hemoglobin difference between black and white women with comparable iron status: justification for race-specific anemia criteria. *American Journal of Clinical Nutrition.* 1994;60(1): 117–121.

10 Tirlapur VG, Gicheru K, Charalambous BM et al. Packed cell volume, haemoglobin, and oxygen saturation changes in healthy smokers and non-smokers. *Thorax.* 1983;38(10):785–787.

11 Silverberg DS, Blum M, Agbaria Z et al. The effect of i.v. iron alone or in combination with low-dose erythropoietin in the rapid correction of anemia of chronic renal failure in the predialysis period. *Clinical Nephrology.* 2001;55(3):212–219.

12 Department of Health. *The National Service Framework for Renal Services. Part One: Dialysis and Transplantation.* London: Department of Health, 2004.

13 Department of Health. *National Service Framework for Renal Services. Part Two: chronic kidney disease, acute renal failure and end of life care.* London: Department of Health, 2005.

14 Stevens ME, Summerfield GP, Hall AA et al. Cost benefits of low dose subcutaneous erythropoietin in patients with anaemia of end stage renal disease. *British Medical Journal.* 1992;304(6825):474–477.

15 Renal Association. *UK Renal Registry Annual Report* (seventh). Renal Association, 2004.

16 De Lusignan S, Stevens PE, O'Donoghue D et al. Identifying patients with chronic kidney disease from general practice computer records. *Family Practice.* 2005;22(3):234–241.

17 Lindeman RD, Tobin JD, Shock NW. Association between blood pressure and the rate of decline in renal function with age. *Kidney International.* 1984;26(6):861–868.

18 Fliser D, Franek E, Ritz E. Renal function in the elderly – is the dogma of an inexorable decline of renal function correct? *Nephrology Dialysis Transplantation.* 1997;12(8):1553–1555.

19 Kasiske BL. Relationship between vascular disease and age-associated changes in the human kidney. *Kidney International.* 1987;31(5):1153–1159.

20 Fliser D, Klimm HD, Horner D et al. Proteinuria as a function of hypertension and age. *Contributions to Nephrology.* 1993;105:25–32.

21 Rahman M, Brown CD, Coresh J et al. The prevalence of reduced glomerular filtration rate in older hypertensive patients and its association with cardiovascular disease: a report from the Antihypertensive and Lipid-Lowering Treatment to Prevent Heart Attack Trial. *Archives of Internal Medicine.* 2004;164(9): 969–976.

22 Coresh J, Astor BC, Greene T et al. Prevalence of chronic kidney disease and decreased kidney function in the adult US population: Third National Health and Nutrition Examination Survey. *American Journal of Kidney Diseases.* 2003;41(1):1–12.

23 John R, Webb M, Young A et al. Unreferred Chronic Kidney Disease: A Longitudinal Study. *American Journal of Kidney Diseases.* 2004;43(5):825–835.

24 Kojima K, Totsuka Y. Anemia due to reduced serum erythropoietin concentration in non-uremic diabetic patients. *Diabetes Research & Clinical Practice.* 1995;27(3):229–233.

25 Ishimura E, Nishizawa Y, Okuno S et al. Diabetes mellitus increases the severity of anemia in non-dialyzed patients with renal failure. *Journal of Nephrology.* 1998;11(2):83–86.

26 Bosman DR, Winkler AS, Marsden JT et al. Anemia with erythropoietin deficiency occurs early in diabetic nephropathy. *Diabetes Care.* 2001;24(3):495–499.

27 Thomas MC, MacIsaac RJ, Tsalamandris C et al. Unrecognized anemia in patients with diabetes: a cross-sectional survey. *Diabetes Care.* 2003;26(4):1164–1169.

28 Thomas MC, MacIsaac RJ, Tsalamandris C et al. The burden of anaemia in Type 2 diabetes and the role of nephropathy: a cross-sectional audit. *Nephrology Dialysis Transplantation.* 2004;19(7):1792–1797.

29 Thomas MC, Cooper ME, Tsalamandris C et al. Anemia with impaired erythropoietin response in diabetic patients. *Archives of Internal Medicine.* 2005;165(4):466–469.

30 El Achkar TM, Ohmit SE, McCullough PA et al. Higher prevalence of anemia with diabetes mellitus in moderate kidney insufficiency: The Kidney Early Evaluation Program. *Kidney International.* 2005;67(4): 1483–1488.

31 Guyatt GH, Patterson C, Ali M et al. Diagnosis of iron-deficiency anemia in the elderly. *American Journal of Medicine.* 1990;88(3):205–209.

32 Patterson C, Guyatt GH, Singer J et al. Iron deficiency anemia in the elderly: the diagnostic process. *Canadian Medical Association Journal.* 1991;144(4):435–440.

33 Joosten E, Pelemans W, Hiele M et al. Prevalence and causes of anaemia in a geriatric hospitalized population. *Gerontology.* 1992;38(1–2):111–117.

34 National Institute for Clinical Excellence. *The guideline development process: an overview for stakeholders, the public and the NHS.* London: NICE, 2004.

35 National Collaborating Centre for Chronic Conditions. *Methodology Pack.* 2006.

36 National Institute for Clinical Excellence. *Delivering Quality in the NHS 2004.* Oxford: Radcliffe Medical Press, 2004.

37 Portoles J, Torralbo A, Martin P et al. Cardiovascular effects of recombinant human erythropoietin in predialysis patients. *American Journal of Kidney Diseases.* 1997;29(4):541–548.

38 Ifudu O, Uribarri J, Rajwani I et al. Low hematocrit may connote a malnutrition/inflammation syndrome in hemodialysis patients. *Dialysis & Transplantation.* 2002;31(12).

39 Wolfe RA, Hulbert-Shearon TE, Ashby VB et al. Improvements in dialysis patient mortality are associated with improvements in urea reduction ratio and hematocrit, 1999 to 2002. *American Journal of Kidney Diseases.* 2005;45(1):127–135.

40 Weiner DE, Tighiouart H, Vlagopoulos PT et al. Effects of anemia and left ventricular hypertrophy on cardiovascular disease in patients with chronic kidney disease. *Journal of the American Society of Nephrology.* 2005;16(6):1803–1810.

41 Hayashi T, Suzuki A, Shoji T et al. Cardiovascular effect of normalizing the hematocrit level during erythropoietin therapy in predialysis patients with chronic renal failure. *American Journal of Kidney Diseases.* 2000;35(2):250–256.

42   Silberberg J, Racine N, Barre P et al. Regression of left ventricular hypertrophy in dialysis patients following correction of anemia with recombinant human erythropoietin. *Canadian Journal of Cardiology.* 1990;6(1):1–4.

43   Metry G, Wikstrom B, Valind S et al. Effect of normalization of hematocrit on brain circulation and metabolism in hemodialysis patients. *Journal of the American Society of Nephrology.* 1999;10(4):854–863.

44   Moreno F, Aracil FJ, Perez R et al. Controlled study on the improvement of quality of life in elderly hemodialysis patients after correcting end-stage renal disease-related anemia with erythropoietin. *American Journal of Kidney Diseases.* 1996;27(4):548–556.

45   Ma JZ, Ebben J, Xia H et al. Hematocrit level and associated mortality in hemodialysis patients. *Journal of the American Society of Nephrology.* 1999;10(3):610–619.

46   Collins AJ, Li S, St Peter W et al. Death, hospitalization, and economic associations among incident hemodialysis patients with hematocrit values of 36 to 39%. *Journal of the American Society of Nephrology.* 2001;12(11):2465–2473.

47   Li S, Collins AJ. Association of hematocrit value with cardiovascular morbidity and mortality in incident hemodialysis patients. *Kidney International.* 2004;65(2):626–633.

48   Levin A, Thompson CR, Ethier J et al. Left ventricular mass index increase in early renal disease: impact of decline in hemoglobin. *American Journal of Kidney Diseases.* 1999;34(1):125–134.

49   Moreno F, Sanz-Guajardo D, Lopez-Gomez JM et al. Increasing the hematocrit has a beneficial effect on quality of life and is safe in selected hemodialysis patients. Spanish Cooperative Renal Patients Quality of Life Study Group of the Spanish Society of Nephrology. *Journal of the American Society of Nephrology.* 2000;11(2):335–342.

50   Djamali A, Becker YT, Simmons WD et al. Increasing hematocrit reduces early posttransplant cardiovascular risk in diabetic transplant recipients. *Transplantation.* 2003;76(5):816–820.

51   Jones M, Schenkel B, Just J. Epoetin alfa's effect on left ventricular hypertrophy and subsequent mortality. *International Journal of Cardiology.* 2005;100(2):253–265.

52   Lee SY, Lee H-J, Kim Y-K et al. Neurocognitive function and quality of life in relation to hematocrit levels in chronic hemodialysis patients. *Journal of Psychosomatic Research.* 2004;57(1):5–10.

53   Stevens P, O'Donoghue D, Lameire N. Anaemia in patients with diabetes: unrecognized, undetected and untreated? *Current Medical Research & Opinion.* 2003;195:395–401.

54   Tielemans CL, Lenclud CM, Wens R et al. Critical role of iron overload in the increased susceptibility of haemodialysis patients to bacterial infections. Beneficial effects of desferrioxamine. *Nephrology Dialysis Transplantation.* 1989;4(10):883–887.

55   Astor BC, Muntner P, Levin A et al. Association of kidney function with anemia: the Third National Health and Nutrition Examination Survey (1988–1994). *Archives of Internal Medicine.* 2002;162(12):1401–1408.

56   Hsu CY, Bates DW, Kuperman GJ et al. Relationship between hematocrit and renal function in men and women. *Kidney International.* 2001;59(2):725–731.

57   McClellan W, Aronoff SL, Bolton WK et al. The prevalence of anemia in patients with chronic kidney disease. *Current Medical Research & Opinion.* 2004;20(9):1501–1510.

58   Kazmi WH, Kausz AT, Khan S et al. Anemia: An early complication of chronic renal insufficiency. *American Journal of Kidney Diseases.* 2001;38(4):803–812.

59   Fivush BA, Jabs K, Neu AM et al. Chronic renal insufficiency in children and adolescents: the 1996 annual report of NAPRTCS. North American Pediatric Renal Transplant Cooperative Study. *Pediatric Nephrology.* 1998;12(4):328–337.

60   Kalantar-Zadeh K, Hoffken B, Wunsch H et al. Diagnosis of iron deficiency anemia in renal failure patients during the post-erythropoietin era. *American Journal of Kidney Diseases.* 1995;26(2):292–299.

61   Cullen P, Soffker J, Hopfl M et al. Hypochromic red cells and reticulocyte haemoglobin content as markers of iron-deficient erythropoiesis in patients undergoing chronic haemodialysis. *Nephrology Dialysis Transplantation.* 1999;14(3):659–665.

62 Fernandez-Rodriguez AM, Guindeo-Casasus MC, Molero-Labarta T et al. Diagnosis of iron deficiency in chronic renal failure. *American Journal of Kidney Diseases.* 1999;34(3):508–513.

63 Fishbane S, Lynn RI. The utility of zinc protoporphyrin for predicting the need for intravenous iron therapy in hemodialysis patients. *American Journal of Kidney Diseases.* 1995;25(3):426–432.

64 Fishbane S, Galgano C, Langley RC, Jr. et al. Reticulocyte hemoglobin content in the evaluation of iron status of hemodialysis patients. *Kidney International.* 1997;52(1):217–222.

65 Low CL, Bailie GR, Eisele G. Sensitivity and specificity of transferrin saturation and serum ferritin as markers of iron status after intravenous iron dextran in hemodialysis patients. *Renal Failure.* 1997;19(6):781–788.

66 Tessitore N, Solero GP, Lippi G et al. The role of iron status markers in predicting response to intravenous iron in haemodialysis patients on maintenance erythropoietin. *Nephrology Dialysis Transplantation.* 2001;16(7):1416–1423.

67 Kaneko Y, Miyazaki S, Hirasawa Y et al. Transferrin saturation vs reticulocyte hemoglobin content for iron deficiency in Japanese hemodialysis patients. *Kidney International.* 2003;63:1086–1093.

68 Kaufman JS, Reda DJ, Fye CL et al. Diagnostic value of iron indices in hemodialysis patients receiving epoetin. *Kidney International.* 2001;60(1):300–308.

69 Blagg C. EPO – one year later. Part II. Balancing the costs and benefits. *Nephrology News & Issues.* 1990;4(6):22–38.

70 Radtke HW, Claussner A, Erbes PM. Serum erythropoietin concentration in chronic renal failure: Relationship to degree of anemia and excretory renal function. *Blood.* 1979;54(4):877–884.

71 Aikhionbare HA, Winterborn MW, Gyde OH. Erythropoietin in children with chronic renal failure on dialytic and non-dialytic therapy. *International Journal of Pediatric Nephrology.* 1987;8(1):9–14.

72 Fehr T, Ammann P, Garzoni D et al. Interpretation of erythropoietin levels in patients with various degrees of renal insufficiency and anemia. *Kidney International.* 2004;66(3):1206–1211.

73 Muller Wiefel DE, Scharer K. Serum erythropoietin levels in children with chronic renal failure. *Kidney International.* 1983;24(Suppl 15)

74 Eckardt KU, Hartmann W, Vetter U et al. Serum immunoreactive erythropoietin of children in health and disease. *European Journal of Pediatrics.* 1990;149(7):459–464.

75 Chandra M, Clemons GK, McVicar MI. Relation of serum erythropoietin levels to renal excretory function: Evidence for lowered set point for erythropoietin production in chronic renal failure. *Journal of Pediatrics.* 1988;113(6):1015–1021.

76 Craig KJ, Williams JD, Riley SG et al. Anemia and diabetes in the absence of nephropathy. *Diabetes Care.* 2005;28(5):1118–1123.

77 Besarab A, Amin N, Ahsan M et al. Optimization of epoetin therapy with intravenous iron therapy in hemodialysis patients. *Journal of the American Society of Nephrology.* 2000;11(3):530–538.

78 Sepandj F, Jindal K, West M et al. Economic appraisal of maintenance parenteral iron administration in treatment of anaemia in chronic haemodialysis patients. *Nephrology Dialysis Transplantation.* 1996;11(2):319–322.

79 Giancaspro V, Nuzziello M, Pallotta G et al. Intravenous ascorbic acid in hemodialysis patients with functional iron deficiency: a clinical trial. *Journal of Nephrology.* 2000;13(6):444–449.

80 Taji Y, Morimoto T, Okada K et al. Effects of intravenous ascorbic acid on erythropoiesis and quality of life in unselected hemodialysis patients. *Journal of Nephrology.* 2004;17(4):537–543.

81 Ono K, Hisasue Y. Is folate supplementation necessary in hemodialysis patients on erythropoietin therapy. *Clinical Nephrology.* 1992;38(5):290–292.

82 Caruso U, Leone L, Cravotto E et al. Effects of L-carnitine on anemia in aged hemodialysis patients treated with recombinant human erythropoietin: A pilot study. *Dialysis & Transplantation.* 1998;27(8):498–506.

83 Labonia WD. L-carnitine effects on anemia in hemodialyzed patients treated with erythropoietin. *American Journal of Kidney Diseases.* 1995;26(5):757–764.

84 Kletzmayr J, Mayer G, Legenstein E et al. Anemia and carnitine supplementation in hemodialyzed patients. *Kidney International.* 1999;69:S93–106.

85 Semeniuk J, Shalansky KF, Taylor N et al. Evaluation of the effect of intravenous l-carnitine on quality of life in chronic hemodialysis patients. *Clinical Nephrology.* 2000;54(6):470–477.

86 Lilien MR, Duran M, Quak JM et al. Oral L-carnitine does not decrease erythropoietin requirement in pediatric dialysis. *Pediatric Nephrology.* 2000;15(1–2):17–20.

87 Tarng DC, Huang TP. A parallel, comparative study of intravenous iron vs intravenous ascorbic acid for erythropoietin-hyporesponsive anaemia in haemodialysis patients with iron overload. *Nephrology Dialysis Transplantation.* 1998;13(11):2867–2872.

88 Tarng DC, Wei YH, Huang TP et al. Intravenous ascorbic acid as an adjuvant therapy for recombinant erythropoietin in hemodialysis patients with hyperferritinemia. *Kidney International.* 1999;55(6): 2477–2486.

89 Sezer S, Ozdemir FN, Yakupoglu U et al. Intravenous ascorbic acid administration for erythropoietin-hyporesponsive anemia in iron loaded hemodialysis patients. *Artificial Organs.* 2002;26(4):366–370.

90 Keven K. Randomized, crossover study of the effect of vitamin C on EPO response in hemodialysis patients. *American Journal of Kidney Diseases.* 2003;41(6):1233–1239.

91 Nemeth I, Turi S, Haszon I et al. Vitamin E alleviates the oxidative stress of erythropoietin in uremic children on hemodialysis. *Pediatric Nephrology.* 2000;14(1):13–17.

92 Klemm A. Is folate and vitamin B12 supplementation necessary in chronic hemodialysis patients with EPO treatment? *Clinical Nephrology.* 1994;42(5):343–345.

93 Hurot JM, Cucherat M, Haugh M et al. Effects of L-carnitine supplementation in maintenance hemodialysis patients: a systematic review. *Journal of the American Society of Nephrology.* 2002;13(3):708–714.

94 Topaloglu R, Celiker A, Saatci U et al. Effect of carnitine supplementation on cardiac function in hemodialyzed children. *Acta Paediatrica Japonica.* 1998;40(1):26–29.

95 Matsumoto Y, Amano I, Hirose S et al. Effects of L-carnitine supplementation on renal anemia in poor responders to erythropoietin. *Blood Purification.* 2001;19(1):24–32.

96 Romagnoli GF, Naso A, Carraro G et al. Beneficial effects of L-carnitine in dialysis patients with impaired left ventricular function: an observational study. *Current Medical Research & Opinion.* 2002;18(3): 172–175.

97 Sotirakopoulos N, Athanasiou G, Tsitsios T et al. The influence of L-carnitine supplementation on hematocrit and hemoglobin levels in patients with end stage renal failure on CAPD. *Renal Failure.* 2002;24(4):505–510.

98 DeGowin RL, Lavender AR, Forland M et al. Erythropoiesis and erythropoietin in patients with chronic renal failure treated with hemodialysis and testosterone. *Annals of Internal Medicine.* 1970;72(6):913–918.

99 Fried W, Jonasson O, Lang G et al. The hematologic effect of androgen in uremic patients. Study of packed cell volume and erythropoietin responses. *Annals of Internal Medicine.* 1973;79(6):823–827.

100 Hendler ED, Goffinet JA, Ross S et al. Controlled study of androgen therapy in anemia of patients on maintenance hemodialysis. *New England Journal of Medicine.* 1974;291(20):1046–1051.

101 Williams JS, Stein JH, Ferris TF. Nandrolone decanoate therapy for patients receiving hemodialysis. A controlled study. *Archives of Internal Medicine.* 1974;134(2):289–292.

102 Cattran DC, Fenton SS, Wilson DR et al. A controlled trial of nondrolone decanoate in the treatment of uremic anemia. *Kidney International.* 1977;12(6):430–437.

103 Naik RB, Gibbons AR, Gyde OH et al. Androgen trial in renal anaemia. *Proceedings of the European Dialysis & Transplant Association.* 1978;15:136–143.

104 Navarro JF, Mora C, Macia M et al. Randomized prospective comparison between erythropoietin and androgens in CAPD patients. *Kidney International.* 2002;61(4):1537–1544.

105 Gaughan WJ, Liss KA, Dunn SR et al. A 6-month study of low-dose recombinant human erythropoietin alone and in combination with androgens for the treatment of anemia in chronic hemodialysis patients. *American Journal of Kidney Diseases.* 1997;30(4):495–500.

106 Ballal SH, Domoto DT, Polack DC et al. Androgens potentiate the effects of erythropoietin in the treatment of anemia of end-stage renal disease. *American Journal of Kidney Diseases.* 1991;17(1):29–33.

107 Teruel JL, Marcen R, Navarro-Antolin J et al. Androgen vs erythropoietin for the treatment of anemia in hemodialyzed patients: a prospective study. *Journal of the American Society of Nephrology.* 1996;7(1): 140–144.

108 Teruel JL, Aguilera A, Marcen R et al. Androgen therapy for anaemia of chronic renal failure. *Scandinavian Journal of Urology & Nephrology.* 1996;30(5):403–408.

109 Lee MS, Ahn SH, Song JH. Effects of adjuvant androgen on anemia and nutritional parameters in chronic hemodialysis patients using low-dose recombinant human erythropoietin. *Korean Journal of Internal Medicine.* 2002;17(3):167–173.

110 Berns JS, Rudnick MR, Cohen RM. A controlled trial of recombinant human erythropoietin and nandrolone decanoate in the treatment of anemia in patients on chronic hemodialysis. *Clinical Nephrology.* 1992;37(5):264–267.

111 Gascon A, Belvis JJ, Berisa F et al. Nandrolone decanoate is a good alternative for the treatment of anemia in elderly male patients on hemodialysis. *Geriatric Nephrology & Urology.* 1999;9(2):67–72.

112 Turner G, Brown RC, Silver A et al. Renal insufficiency and secondary hyperparathyroidism in elderly patients. *Annals of Clinical Biochemistry.* 1991;28 (Pt 4):321–326.

113 Reichel H, Deibert B, Schmidt-Gayk H et al. Calcium metabolism in early chronic renal failure: implications for the pathogenesis of hyperparathyroidism. *Nephrology Dialysis Transplantation.* 1991;6(3): 162–169.

114 St John A, Thomas MB, Davies CP et al. Determinants of intact parathyroid hormone and free 1,25-dihydroxyvitamin D levels in mild and moderate renal failure. *Nephron.* 1992;61(4):422–427.

115 De Boer IH, Gorodetskaya I, Young B et al. The severity of secondary hyperparathyroidism in chronic renal insufficiency is GFR-dependent, race-dependent, and associated with cardiovascular disease. *Journal of the American Society of Nephrology.* 2002;13(11):2762–2769.

116 Lee CT, Chou FF, Chang HW et al. Effects of parathyroidectomy on iron homeostasis and erythropoiesis in hemodialysis patients with severe hyperparathyroidism. *Blood Purification.* 2003;21(6):369–375.

117 Lin CL, Hung CC, Yang CT et al. Improved anemia and reduced erythropoietin need by medical or surgical intervention of secondary hyperparathyroidism in hemodialysis patients. *Renal Failure.* 2004; 26(3):289–295.

118 Goicoechea M, Vazquez MI, Ruiz MA et al. Intravenous calcitriol improves anaemia and reduces the need for erythropoietin in haemodialysis patients. *Nephron.* 1998;78(1):23–27.

119 Yasunaga C, Matsuo K, Yanagida T et al. Early effects of parathyroidectomy on erythropoietin production in secondary hyperparathyroidism. *American Journal of Surgery.* 2002;183(2):199–204.

120 Albitar S, Genin R, Fen-Chong M et al. High-dose alfacalcidol improves anaemia in patients on haemodialysis. *Nephrology Dialysis Transplantation.* 1997;12(3):514–518.

121 Coen G, Calabria S, Bellinghieri G et al. Parathyroidectomy in chronic renal failure: short- and long-term results on parathyroid function, blood pressure and anemia. *Nephron.* 2001;88(2):149–155.

122 Rault R, Magnone M. The effect of parathyroidectomy on hematocrit and erythropoietin dose in patients on hemodialysis. *ASAIO Journal.* 1996;42(5):M901–903.

123 Fujita Y, Inoue S, Horiguchi S et al. Excessive level of parathyroid hormone may induce the reduction of recombinant human erythropoietin effect on renal anemia. *Mineral & Electrolyte Metabolism.* 1995; 21(1–3):50–54.

124 Nazem AK, Mako J. The effect of calcitriol on renal anaemia in patients undergoing long-term dialysis. *International Urology & Nephrology.* 1997;29(1):119–127.

125 Barbour GL. Effect of parathyroidectomy on anemia in chronic renal failure. *Archives of Internal Medicine.* 1979;139(8):889–891.

126 Podjarny E, Rathaus M, Korzets Z et al. Is anemia of chronic renal failure related to secondary hyperparathyroidism? *Archives of Internal Medicine.* 1981;141(4):453–455.

127 Zingraff J, Drueke T, Marie P et al. Anemia and secondary hyperparathyroidism. *Archives of Internal Medicine.* 1978;138(11):1650–1652.

128 Urena P, Eckardt KU, Sarfati E et al. Serum erythropoietin and erythropoiesis in primary and secondary hyperparathyroidism: effect of parathyroidectomy. *Nephron.* 1991;59(3):384–393.

129 Renal Association and Royal College of Physicians. *Treatment of adults and children with renal failure. Recommended standards and audit measures.* 2003.

130 Massry SG, Coburn JW, Chertow GM et al. K/DOQI clinical practice guidelines for bone metabolism and disease in chronic kidney disease. *American Journal of Kidney Diseases.* 2003;42(4 Suppl 3):i–S201.

131 Anon. European Best Practice Guidelines for Haemodialysis. *Nephrology Dialysis Transplantation.* 2002;17 Suppl 7:1–111.

132 Muirhead N, Churchill DN, Goldstein M et al. Comparison of subcutaneous and intravenous recombinant human erythropoietin for anemia in hemodialysis patients with significant comorbid disease. *American Journal of Nephrology.* 1992;12:303–310.

133 Granolleras C, Leskopf W, Shaldon S et al. Experience of pain after subcutaneous administration of different preparations of recombinant human erythropoietin: A randomized, double-blind crossover study. *Clinical Nephrology.* 1991;36(6):294–298.

134 Wazny LD, Stojimirovic BB, Heidenheim P et al. Factors influencing erythropoietin compliance in peritoneal dialysis patients. *American Journal of Kidney Diseases.* 2002;40(3):623–628.

135 Nicoletta P, Bernardini J, Dacko C et al. Compliance with subcutaneous erythropoietin in peritoneal dialysis patients. *Advances in Peritoneal Dialysis.* 2000;16:90–92.

136 Mahon A, Docherty B. Renal anaemia – the patient experience. *Edtna-Erca Journal.* 2004;30(1):34–37.

137 Ashcroft DM, Clark CM, Gorman SP. Shared care: A study of patients' experiences with erythropoietin. *International Journal of Pharmacy Practice.* 1998;6(3):145–149.

138 National Kidney Federation. *National Kidney Federation Anaemia Survey.* 2004.

139 Bailie GR, Plitnick R, Eisele G et al. Experience with subcutaneous erythropoietin in CAPD patients. *Advances in Peritoneal Dialysis.* 1991;7:292–295.

140 Roche A. *The Health Education Needs of Patients who require Erythropoetin Therapy : MA Thesis De Montfort University.* 2005.

141 Cody J, Daly C, Campbell M et al. Recombinant human erythropoietin for chronic renal failure anaemia in predialysis patients. *The Cochrane Library.* 2004;(4)

142 Anon. Association between recombinant human erythropoietin and quality of life and exercise capacity of patients receiving haemodialysis. Canadian Erythropoietin Study Group. *British Medical Journal.* 1990;300(6724):573–578.

143 Nissenson AR, Korbet S, Faber M et al. Multicenter trial of erythropoietin in patients on peritoneal dialysis. *Journal of the American Society of Nephrology.* 1995;5(7):1517–1529.

144 Churchill DN, Muirhead N, Goldstein M et al. Effect of recombinant human erythropoietin on hospitalization of hemodialysis patients. *Clinical Nephrology.* 1995;43(3):184–188.

145 Powe NR, Griffiths R, I, Watson AJ et al. Effect of recombinant erythropoietin on hospital admissions, readmissions, length of stay, and costs of dialysis patients. *Journal of the American Society of Nephrology.* 1994;4(7):1455–1465.

146 Bahlmann J, Schoter KH, Scigalla P et al. Morbidity and mortality in hemodialysis patients with and without erythropoietin treatment: a controlled study. *Contributions to Nephrology.* 1991;88:90–106.

147 Leese B, Hutton J, Maynard A. A comparison of the costs and benefits of recombinant human erythropoietin (epoetin) in the treatment of chronic renal failure in 5 European countries. *Pharmacoeconomics.* 1992;1(5):346–356.

148 Remak E, Hutton J, Jones M et al. Changes in cost-effectiveness over time. *European Journal of Health Economics.* 2003;4(2):115–121.

149 Moran LJ, Carey P, Johnson CA. Cost-effectiveness of epoetin alfa therapy for anemia of end-stage renal disease. *American Journal of Hospital Pharmacy.* 1992;49(6):1451–1454.

150 Opelz G, Sengar DP, Mickey MR et al. Effect of blood transfusions on subsequent kidney transplants. *Transplantation Proceedings.* 1973;5(1):253–259.

151 Opelz G. Improved kidney graft survival in nontransfused recipients. *Transplantation Proceedings.* 1987;19(1 Pt 1):149–152.

152 Flye MW, Burton K, Mohanakumar T et al. Donor-specific transfusions have long-term beneficial effects for human renal allografts. *Transplantation.* 1995;60(12):1395–1401.

153 Opelz G, Vanrenterghem Y, Kirste G et al. Prospective evaluation of pretransplant blood transfusions in cadaver kidney recipients. *Transplantation.* 1997;63(7):964–967.

154 Chavers BM, Sullivan EK, Tejani A et al. Pre-transplant blood transfusion and renal allograft outcome: a report of the North American Pediatric Renal Transplant Cooperative Study. *Pediatric Transplantation.* 1997;1(1):22–28.

155 Soosay A, O'Neill D, Counihan A et al. Causes of sensitisation in patients awaiting renal transplantation in Ireland. *Irish Medical Journal.* 2003;96(4):109–112.

156 Crowley JP, Valeri CR, Metzger JB et al. Lymphocyte subpopulations in long-term dialysis patients: A case-controlled study of the effects of blood transfusion. *Transfusion.* 1990;30(7):644–647.

157 D'Apice AJF, Tait BD. An elective transfusion policy: Sensitization rates, patient transplantability, and transplant outcome. *Transplantation.* 1982;33(2):191–195.

158 Nanishi F, Inenaga T, Onoyama K. Immune alterations in hemodialyzed patients. I. Effect of blood transfusion on T-lymphocyte subpopulations in hemodialyzed patients. *Journal of Clinical & Laboratory Immunology.* 1986;19(4):167–174.

159 Bender BS, Curtis JL, Nagel JE et al. Analysis of immune status of hemodialyzed adults: association with prior transfusions. *Kidney International.* 1984;26(4):436–443.

160 Deenitchina SS, Ando T, Okuda S et al. Influence of recombinant human erythropoietin and blood transfusions on the composition of lymphocyte populations in hemodialyzed patients. *Current Therapeutic Research, Clinical & Experimental.* 1995;56(11):1185–1200.

161 Deierhoi MH, Shroyer TW, Hudson SL et al. Sustained high panel reactive antibody levels in highly sensitized patients: significance of continued transfusions. *Transplantation Proceedings.* 1989;21(1 Pt 1): 771–772.

162 Chapman JF, Elliott C, Knowles SM et al. Guidelines for compatibility procedures in blood transfusion laboratories. *Transfusion Medicine.* 2004;14(1):59–73.

163 Nissenson AR, Swan SK, Lindberg JS et al. Randomized, controlled trial of darbepoetin alfa for the treatment of anemia in hemodialysis patients. *American Journal of Kidney Diseases.* 2002;40(1):110–118.

164 Locatelli F, Olivares J, Walker R et al. Novel erythropoiesis stimulating protein for treatment of anemia in chronic renal insufficiency. *Kidney International.* 2001;60(2):741–747.

165 Tolman C, Richardson D, Bartlett C et al. Structured Conversion from thrice weekly to weekly erythropoietic regimens using a computerized decision-support system: a randomized clinical trial. *Journal of the American Society of Nephrology.* 2005;16(5):1463–1470.

166 Morreale A, Plowman B, DeLattre M et al. Clinical and economic comparison of epoetin alfa and darbepoetin alfa. *Current Medical Research & Opinion.* 2004;20(3):381–395.

167 Gouva C, Nikolopoulos P, Ioannidis JP et al. Treating anemia early in renal failure patients slows the decline of renal function: a randomized controlled trial. *Kidney International.* 66;753–760. 2004.

168 Roger SD, McMahon LP, Clarkson A et al. Effects of early and late intervention with epoetin alpha on left ventricular mass among patients with chronic kidney disease (stage 3 or 4): results of a randomized clinical trial. *Journal of the American Society of Nephrology.* 15;148–156. 2004.

169 Bennett L. The anaemia research nurse in effective multidisciplinary management of patients on erythropoietin. *Edtna-Erca Journal.* 1998;24(3):38–39.

170 De Schoenmakere G, Lameire N, Dhondt A et al. The haematopoietic effect of recombinant human erythropoietin in haemodialysis is independent of the mode of administration (i.v. or s.c.). *Nephrology Dialysis Transplantation.* 1998;13(7):1770–1775.

171 Johnson CA, Wakeen M, Taylor III CA et al. Comparison of intraperitoneal and subcutaneous epoetin alfa in peritoneal dialysis patients. *Peritoneal Dialysis International.* 1999;19(6):578–582.

172 Kaufman JS, Reda DJ, Fye CL et al. Subcutaneous compared with intravenous epoetin in patients receiving hemodialysis. Department of Veterans Affairs Cooperative Study Group on Erythropoietin in Hemodialysis Patients. *New England Journal of Medicine.* 1998;339(9):578–583.

173 Lai KN, Lui SF, Leung JC et al. Effect of subcutaneous and intraperitoneal administration of recombinant human erythropoietin on blood pressure and vasoactive hormones in patients on continuous ambulatory peritoneal dialysis. *Nephron.* 1991;57(4):394–400.

174 Leikis MJ, Kent AB, Becker GJ et al. Haemoglobin response to subcutaneous vs intravenous epoetin alfa administration in iron-replete haemodialysis patients. *Nephrology.* 2004;9(3):153–160.

175 Virot JS, Janin G, Guillaumie J et al. Must erythropoietin be injected by the subcutaneous route for every hemodialyzed patient? *American Journal of Kidney Diseases.* 1996;28(3):400–408.

176 Frifelt JJ, Tvedegaard E, Bruun K et al. Efficacy of recombinant human erythropoietin administered subcutaneously to CAPD patients once weekly. *Peritoneal Dialysis International.* 1996;16(6):594–598.

177 Lui SF, Wong KC, Li PK et al. Once weekly vs twice weekly subcutaneous administration of recombinant human erythropoietin in haemodialysis patients. *American Journal of Nephrology.* 1992;12(1–2):55–60.

178 Paganini EP, Eschbach JW, Lazarus JM et al. Intravenous vs subcutaneous dosing of epoetin alfa in hemodialysis patients. *American Journal of Kidney Diseases.* 1995;26(2):331–340.

179 Eidemak I, Friedberg MO, Ladefoged SD et al. Intravenous vs subcutaneous administration of recombinant human erythropoietin in patients on haemodialysis and CAPD. *Nephrology Dialysis Transplantation.* 1992; 7(6):526–529.

180 Lai PC, Wu MS, Huang JY et al. Efficacy of intravenous and subcutaneous erythropoietin in patients on hemodialysis and continuous ambulatory peritoneal dialysis. *Changgeng Yi Xue Za Zhi.* 1994;17(2): 105–112.

181 Pais MJ, Gaspar A, Santana A et al. Subcutaneous recombinant human erythropoietin in hemodialysis and continuous ambulatory peritoneal dialysis. *Peritoneal Dialysis International.* 1993;13(Suppl 2):S541–S543.

182 Navarro JF, Teruel JL, Marcen R et al. Improvement of erythropoietin-induced hypertension in hemodialysis patients changing the administration route. *Scandinavian Journal of Urology & Nephrology.* 1995;29(1):11–14.

183 Frenken LA, van Lier HJ, Gerlag PG et al. Assessment of pain after subcutaneous injection of erythropoietin in patients receiving haemodialysis. *British Medical Journal.* 1991;303(6797):288.

184 Jensen JD, Madsen JK, Jensen LW. Comparison of dose requirement, serum erythropoietin and blood pressure following intravenous and subcutaneous erythropoietin treatment of dialysis patients. IV and s.c. erythropoietin. *European Journal of Clinical Pharmacology.* 1996;50(3):171–177.

185 Nasu T, Mitui H, Shinohara Y et al. Effect of erythropoietin in continuous ambulatory peritoneal dialysis patients: comparison between intravenous and intraperitoneal administration. *Peritoneal Dialysis International.* 1992;12(4):373–377.

186 Stegmayr BG. Better response to s.c. erythropoietin in CAPD than HD patients. *Scandinavian Journal of Urology & Nephrology.* 1997;31(2):183–187.

187 McClellan WM, Frankenfield DL, Wish JB et al. Subcutaneous erythropoietin results in lower dose and equivalent hematocrit levels among adult hemodialysis patients: Results from the 1998 End-Stage Renal Disease Core Indicators Project. *American Journal of Kidney Diseases.* 2001;37(5):E36.

188 Barre P, Reichel H, Suranyi MG et al. Efficacy of once-weekly epoetin alfa. *Clinical Nephrology.* 2004;62(6): 440–448.

189 Barany P, Clyne N, Hylander B et al. Subcutaneous epoetin beta in renal anemia: an open multicenter dose titration study of patients on continuous peritoneal dialysis. *Peritoneal Dialysis International.* 1995;15(1):54–60.

190 Aronoff GR, Duff DR, Sloan RS et al. The treatment of anemia with low-dose recombinant human erythropoietin. *American Journal of Nephrology.* 1990;10(Suppl 2):40–43.

191 Conlon PJ, Kovalik E, Schumm D et al. Normalization of hematocrit in hemodialysis patients with cardiac disease does not increase blood pressure. *Renal Failure.* 2000;22(4):435–444.

192 Albertazzi A, Di Liberato L, Daniele F et al. Efficacy and tolerability of recombinant human erythropoietin treatment in predialysis patients: results of a multicenter study. *International Journal of Artificial Organs.* 1998;21(1):12–18.

193 Aufricht C, Marik JL, Ettenger RB. Subcutaneous recombinant human erythropoietin in chronic renal allograft dysfunction. *Pediatric Nephrology.* 1998;12(1):10–13.

194 Beshara S, Barany P, Gutierrez A et al. Varying intervals of subcutaneous epoetin alfa in hemodialysis patients. *Journal of Nephrology.* 2004;17(4):525–530.

195 Damme-Lombaerts R, Broyer M, Businger J et al. A study of recombinant human erythropoietin in the treatment of anaemia of chronic renal failure in children on haemodialysis. *Pediatric Nephrology.* 1994;8(3):338–342.

196 Faller B, Slingeneyer A, Waller M et al. Daily subcutaneous administration of recombinant human erythropoietin (rhEPO) in peritoneal dialysis patients: a European dose-response study. *Clinical Nephrology.* 1993;40(3):168–175.

197 Walter J, Gal J, Taraba I. The beneficial effect of low initial dose and gradual increase of erythropoietin treatment in hemodialysis patients. *Artificial Organs.* 1995;19(1):76–80.

198 Besarab A, Reyes CM, Hornberger J. Meta-analysis of subcutaneous vs intravenous epoetin in maintenance treatment of anemia in hemodialysis patients. *American Journal of Kidney Diseases.* 2002; 40(3):439–446.

199 Parker KP, Mitch WE, Stivelman JC et al. Safety and efficacy of low-dose subcutaneous erythropoietin in hemodialysis patients. *Journal of the American Society of Nephrology.* 1997;8(2):288–293.

200 Decaudin B, Lemaitre V, Gautier S et al. Epoetin in haemodialysis patients: impact of change from subcutaneous to intravenous routes of administration. *Journal of Clinical Pharmacy & Therapeutics.* 2004; 29(4):325–329.

201 Martin-Holohan A, Curtis KA, Masterson P et al. Conversion of Chronic Hemodialysis Patients from Erythropoietin Alfa to Darbepoetin Alfa. *Hospital Pharmacy.* 2004;39(4):333–337.

202 Strippoli GFM, Craig JC, Manno C et al. Hemoglobin Targets for the Anemia of Chronic Kidney Disease: A Meta-analysis of Randomized, Controlled Trials. *Journal of the American Society of Nephrology.* 2004;15:3154–3165.

203 McMahon LP, Johns JA, McKenzie A et al. Haemodynamic changes and physical performance at comparative levels of haemoglobin after long-term treatment with recombinant erythropoietin. *Nephrology Dialysis Transplantation.* 1992;7(12):1199–1206.

204 McMahon LP, Dawborn JK. Subjective quality of life assessment in hemodialysis patients at different levels of hemoglobin following use of recombinant human erythropoietin. *American Journal of Nephrology.* 1992;12(3):162–169.

205 Parfrey PS, Foley RN, Wittreich BH et al. Double-Blind Comparison of Full and Partial Anemia Correction in Incident Hemodialysis Patients without Symptomatic Heart Disease. *Journal of the American Society of Nephrology.* 2005;16(7):2180–2189.

206 Frank H, Heusser K, Hoffken B et al. Effect of erythropoietin on cardiovascular prognosis parameters in hemodialysis patients. *Kidney International.* 2004;66(2):832–840.

207 Besarab A, Bolton WK, Browne JK et al. The effects of normal as compared with low hematocrit values in patients with cardiac disease who are receiving hemodialysis and epoetin. *New England Journal of Medicine.* 1998;339(9):584–590.

208 Tonelli M, Winkelmayer WC, Jindal KK et al. The cost-effectiveness of maintaining higher hemoglobin targets with erythropoietin in hemodialysis patients. *Kidney International.* 2003;64(1):295–304.

209 Brandt JR, Avner ED, Hickman RO et al. Safety and efficacy of erythropoietin in children with chronic renal failure. *Pediatric Nephrology.* 1999;13(2):143–147.

210 Morris KP, Sharp J, Watson S et al. Non-cardiac benefits of human recombinant erythropoietin in end stage renal failure and anaemia. *Archives of Disease in Childhood.* 1993;69(5):580–586.

211 Morris KP, Skinner JR, Hunter S et al. Short term correction of anaemia with recombinant human erythropoietin and reduction of cardiac output in end stage renal failure. *Archives of Disease in Childhood.* 1993;68(5):644–648.

212 Lacson E Jr, Ofsthun N, Lazarus JM. Effect of variability in anemia management on hemoglobin outcomes in ESRD. *American Journal of Kidney Diseases.* 2003;41(1):111–124.

213 Fishbane S, Berns JS. Hemoglobin cycling in hemodialysis patients treated with recombinant human erythropoietin. *Kidney International.* 2005;68(3):1337–1343.

214 Nakamoto H, Kanno Y, Okada H et al. Erythropoietin resistance in patients on continuous ambulatory peritoneal dialysis. *Advances in Peritoneal Dialysis.* 2004;20:111–116.

215 Odabas AR, Cetinkaya R, Selcuk Y et al. The effect of high dose losartan on erythropoietin resistance in patients undergoing haemodialysis. *Panminerva Medica.* 2003;45(1):59–62.

216 Albitar S, Genin R, Fen-Chong M et al. High dose enalapril impairs the response to erythropoietin treatment in haemodialysis patients. *Nephrology Dialysis Transplantation.* 1998;13(5):1206–1210.

217 Cruz DN, Perazella MA, Abu-Alfa AK et al. Angiotensin-converting enzyme inhibitor therapy in chronic hemodialysis patients: any evidence of erythropoietin resistance? *American Journal of Kidney Diseases.* 1996;28(4):535–540.

218 Richardson D, Bartlett C, Goutcher E et al. Erythropoietin resistance due to dialysate chloramine: the two-way traffic of solutes in haemodialysis. *Nephrology Dialysis Transplantation.* 1999;14(11):2625–2627.

219 Matsumura M, Nomura H, Koni I et al. Angiotensin-converting enzyme inhibitors are associated with the need for increased recombinant human erythropoietin maintenance doses in hemodialysis patients. Risks of Cardiac Disease in Dialysis Patients Study Group. *Nephron.* 1997;77(2):164–168.

220 Abu-Alfa AK, Cruz D, Perazella MA et al. ACE inhibitors do not induce recombinant human erythropoietin resistance in hemodialysis patients. *American Journal of Kidney Diseases.* 2000;35(6): 1076–1082.

221 Neves PL, Trivino J, Casaubon F et al. Elderly patients on chronic hemodialysis: effect of the secondary hyperparathyroidism on the hemoglobin level. *International Urology & Nephrology.* 2002;34(1):147–149.

222 Coladonato JA, Frankenfield DL, Reddan DN et al. Trends in anemia management among US hemodialysis patients. *Journal of the American Society of Nephrology.* 2002;13(5):1288–1295.

223 Yaqub MS, Leiser J, Molitoris BA. Erythropoietin requirements increase following hospitalization in end-stage renal disease patients. *American Journal of Nephrology.* 2001;21(5):390–396.

224 Kalantar-Zadeh K, McAllister CJ, Lehn RS et al. Effect of malnutrition-inflammation complex syndrome on EPO hyporesponsiveness in maintenance hemodialysis patients. *American Journal of Kidney Diseases.* 2003;42(4):761–773.

225 Gunnell J, Yeun JY, Depner TA et al. Acute-phase response predicts erythropoietin resistance in hemodialysis and peritoneal dialysis patients. *American Journal of Kidney Diseases.* 1999;33(1):63–72.

226 Linde T, Sandhagen B, Wikstrom B et al. The required dose of erythropoietin during renal anaemia treatment is related to the degree of impairment in erythrocyte deformability. *Nephrology Dialysis Transplantation.* 1997;12(11):2375–2379.

227 Fluck S, McKane W, Cairns T et al. Chloramine-induced haemolysis presenting as erythropoietin resistance. *Nephrology Dialysis Transplantation.* 1999;14(7):1687–1691.

228 Piccoli A, Puggia RM, Fusaro M et al. A decision analysis comparing three dosage regimens of subcutaneous epoetin in continuous ambulatory peritoneal dialysis. *Pharmacoeconomics.* 1995;7(5): 444–456.

229 NHS Estates. *Satellite Dialysis Unit: Facilities for Renal services.* (53 volume 1). London: TSO, 2004.

230 Kooistra MP, Niemantsverdriet EC, van Es A et al. Iron absorption in erythropoietin-treated haemodialysis patients: effects of iron availability, inflammation and aluminium. *Nephrology Dialysis Transplantation.* 1998;13(1):82–88.

231 Kooistra MP, Marx JJ. The absorption of iron is disturbed in recombinant human erythropoietin-treated peritoneal dialysis patients. *Nephrology Dialysis Transplantation.* 1998;13(10):2578–2582.

232 Skikne BS, Ahluwalia N, Fergusson B et al. Effects of erythropoietin therapy on iron absorption in chronic renal failure. *Journal of Laboratory & Clinical Medicine.* 2000;135(6):452–458.

233 Hsu CY, Mcculloch CE, Curhan GC. Iron status and hemoglobin level in chronic renal insufficiency. *Journal of the American Society of Nephrology.* 2002;13(11):2783–2786.

234 Van Wyck D, Roppolo M, Martinez C et al. A randomized, controlled trial comparing IV iron sucrose to oral iron in anemic patients with nondialysis-dependent CKD. *Kidney International.* 2005;68(6): 2846–2856.

235 Silverberg DS, Iaina A, Peer G et al. Intravenous iron supplementation for the treatment of the anemia of moderate to severe chronic renal failure patients not receiving dialysis. *American Journal of Kidney Diseases.* 1996;27(2):234–238.

236 Anuradha S, Singh NP, Agarwal SK. Total dose infusion iron dextran therapy in predialysis chronic renal failure patients. *Renal Failure.* 2002;24(3):307–313.

237 Mircescu G, Garneata L, Capusa C et al. Intravenous iron supplementation for the treatment of anaemia in pre-dialyzed chronic renal failure patients. *Nephrology Dialysis Transplantation.* 2006;21(1):120–124.

238 Bhowmik D, Modi G, Ray D et al. Total dose iron infusion: safety and efficacy in predialysis patients. *Renal Failure.* 2000;22(1):39–43.

239 Dahdah K, Patrie JT, Bolton WK. Intravenous iron dextran treatment in predialysis patients with chronic renal failure. *American Journal of Kidney Diseases.* 2000;36(4):775–782.

240 Johnson CA, Rosowski E, Zimmerman SW. A prospective open-label study evaluating the efficacy and adverse reactions of the use of Niferex-150 in ESRD patients receiving EPOGEN. *Advances in Peritoneal Dialysis.* 1992;8:444–447.

241 Agarwal R, Davis JL, Hamburger RJ. A trial of two iron-dextran infusion regimens in chronic hemodialysis patients. *Clinical Nephrology.* 2000;54(2):105–111.

242 Warady BA, Kausz A, Lerner G et al. Iron therapy in the pediatric hemodialysis population. *Pediatric Nephrology.* 2004;19(6):655–661.

243 Ruiz-Jaramillo MdlC. Intermittent vs maintenance iron therapy in children on hemodialysis: a randomised study. *Pediatric Nephrology.* 2004;19:77–81.

244 Warady BA, Zobrist RH, Wu J et al. Sodium ferric gluconate complex therapy in anemic children on hemodialysis. *Pediatric Nephrology.* 2005;20(9):1320–1327.

245 Bailie GR, Clark JA, Lane CE et al. Hypersensitivity reactions and deaths associated with intravenous iron preparations. *Nephrol Dial Transplant.* 2005;20(7):1443–1449.

246 Chertow GM, Mason PD, Vaage-Nilsen O et al. On the relative safety of parenteral iron formulations. *Nephrol Dial Transplant.* 2004;19(6):1571–1575.

247 Chertow GM, Mason PD, Vaage-Nilsen O et al. Update on adverse drug events associated with parenteral iron. *Nephrol Dial Transplant.* 2006;21(2):378–382.

248 Fishbane S, Ungureanu VD, Maesaka JK et al. The safety of intravenous iron dextran in hemodialysis patients. *American Journal of Kidney Diseases.* 1996;28(4):529–534.

249 Fletes R, Lazarus JM, Gage J et al. Suspected iron dextran-related adverse drug events in hemodialysis patients. *American Journal of Kidney Diseases.* 2001;37(4):743–749.

250 Walters BA, Van Wyck DB. Benchmarking iron dextran sensitivity: reactions requiring resuscitative medication in incident and prevalent patients. *Nephrology Dialysis Transplantation.* 2005;20(7): 1438–1442.

251 Fishbane S, Frei GL, Maesaka J. Reduction in recombinant human erythropoietin doses by the use of chronic intravenous iron supplementation. *American Journal of Kidney Diseases.* 1995;26(1):41–46.

252 Macdougall I.C., Tucker B. A randomized controlled study of iron supplementation in patients treated with erythropoietin. *Kidney International.* 1996;50(5):1694–1699.

253 Stoves J, Inglis H, Newstead CG. A randomized study of oral vs intravenous iron supplementation in patients with progressive renal insufficiency treated with erythropoietin. *Nephrology Dialysis Transplantation.* 2001;16(5):967–974.

254 Charytan C, Qunibi W, Bailie GR. Comparison of intravenous iron sucrose to oral iron in the treatment of anemic patients with chronic kidney disease not on dialysis. *Nephron Clinical Practice.* 2005;100(3): c55–62.

255 Ahsan N. Infusion of total dose iron vs oral iron supplementation in ambulatory peritoneal dialysis patients: a prospective, cross-over trial. *Advances in Peritoneal Dialysis.* 2000;16:80–84.

256 Macdougall IC, Chandler G, Elston O et al. Beneficial effects of adopting an aggressive intravenous iron policy in a hemodialysis unit. *American Journal of Kidney Diseases.* 1999;34(4 Suppl 2):S40–S46.

257 Besarab A, Kaiser JW, Frinak S. A study of parenteral iron regimens in hemodialysis patients. *American Journal of Kidney Diseases.* 1999;34(1):21–28.

258 Richardson D, Bartlett C, Will EJ. Optimizing erythropoietin therapy in hemodialysis patients. *American Journal of Kidney Diseases.* 2001;38(1):109–117.

259 Silva J, Andrade S, Ventura H et al. Iron supplementation in haemodialysis-practical clinical guidelines. *Nephrology Dialysis Transplantation.* 1998;13(10):2572–2577.

260 Silverberg DS, Blum M, Peer G et al. Intravenous ferric saccharate as an iron supplement in dialysis patients. *Nephron.* 1996;72(3):413–417.

261 Kato A, Hamada M, Suzuki T et al. Effect of weekly or successive iron supplementation on erythropoietin doses in patients receiving hemodialysis. *Nephron.* 2001;89(1):110–112.

262 Saltissi D, Sauvage D, Westhuyzen J. Comparative response to single or divided doses of parenteral iron for functional iron deficiency in hemodialysis patients receiving erythropoietin (EPO). *Clinical Nephrology.* 1998;49(1):45–48.

263 Auerbach M, Winchester J, Wahab A et al. A randomized trial of three iron dextran infusion methods for anemia in EPO-treated dialysis patients. *American Journal of Kidney Diseases.* 1998;31(1):81–86.

264 Akcicek F, Ozkahya M, Cirit M et al. The efficiency of fractionated parenteral iron treatment in CAPD patients. *Advances in Peritoneal Dialysis.* 1997;13:109–112.

265 Macdougall IC, Roche A. Administration of intravenous iron sucrose as a 2-minute push to CKD patients: A prospective evaluation of 2,297 injections. *American Journal of Kidney Diseases.* 2005;46(2):283–289.

266 Feldman HI, Joffe M, Robinson B et al. Administration of parenteral iron and mortality among hemodialysis patients. *Journal of the American Society of Nephrology.* 2004;15(6):1623–1632.

267 Markowitz GS, Kahn GA, Feingold RE et al. An evaluation of the effectiveness of oral iron therapy in hemodialysis patients receiving recombinant human erythropoietin. *Clinical Nephrology.* 1997;48(1): 34–40.

268 Wingard RL, Parker RA, Ismail N et al. Efficacy of oral iron therapy in patients receiving recombinant human erythropoietin. *American Journal of Kidney Diseases.* 1995;25(3):433–439.

269 Driver PS. Cost-effectiveness impact of iron dextran on hemodialysis patients' use of epoetin alfa and blood. *American Journal of Health-System Pharmacy.* 1998;55(4):S12–16.

270 Morgan HE, Gautam M, Geary DF. Maintenance intravenous iron therapy in pediatric hemodialysis patients. *Pediatric Nephrology.* 2001;16(10):779–783.

271 Bhandari S, Brownjohn A, Turney J. Effective utilization of erythropoietin with intravenous iron therapy. *Journal of Clinical Pharmacy & Therapeutics.* 1998;23(1):73–78.

272 Park L, Uhthoff T, Tierney M et al. Effect of an intravenous iron dextran regimen on iron stores, hemoglobin, and erythropoietin requirements in hemodialysis patients. *American Journal of Kidney Diseases.* 1998;31(5):835–840.

273 Senger JM, Weiss RJ. Hematologic and erythropoietin responses to iron dextran in the hemodialysis environment. *Anna Journal.* 1996;23(3):319–323.

274 St Peter WL, Lambrecht LJ, Macres M. Randomized cross-over study of adverse reactions and cost implications of intravenous push compared with infusion of iron dextran in hemodialysis patients. *American Journal of Kidney Diseases.* 1996;28(4):523–528.

275 Jones CH, Richardson D, Ayers S et al. Percentage hypochromic red cells and the response to intravenous iron therapy in anaemic haemodialysis patients. *Nephrology Dialysis Transplantation.* 1998;13(11):2873–2876.

276 Tenbrock K, Muller-Berghaus J, Michalk D et al. Intravenous iron treatment of renal anemia in children on hemodialysis. *Pediatric Nephrology*. 1999;1323(7):580–582.

277 Jonnalagadda V, Bloom EJ, Raja RM. Importance of iron saturation for erythropoietin responsiveness in chronic peritoneal dialysis. *Advances in Peritoneal Dialysis*. 1997;13(23):113–115.

278 Ifudu O, Friedman EA. Economic implications of inadequate response to erythropoietin in patients with end-stage renal disease. *Dialysis & Transplantation*. 1997;26(10):664–669.

279 Anon. European best practice guidelines for the management of anemia in patients with chronic renal failure. *Nephrology Dialysis Transplantation*. 1999;14(Suppl 5):1–50.

280 Casadevall N, Nataf J, Viron B et al. Pure red-cell aplasia and antierythropoietin antibodies in patients treated with recombinant erythropoietin. *New England Journal of Medicine*. 2002;346(7):469–475.

281 Tarng DC, Huang TP. Recombinant human erythropoietin resistance in iron-replete hemodialysis patients: role of aluminum toxicity. *American Journal of Nephrology*. 1998;18(1):1–8.

282 Sirken G, Kung s.c., Raja R. Decreased erythropoietin requirements in maintenance hemodialysis patients with statin therapy. *ASAIO Journal*. 2003;49(4):422–425.

283 Barany P, Divino Filho JC, Bergstrom J. High C-reactive protein is a strong predictor of resistance to erythropoietin in hemodialysis patients. *American Journal of Kidney Diseases*. 1997;29(4):565–568.

284 Sezer S, Kulah E, Ozdemir FN et al. Clinical consequences of intermittent elevation of C-reactive protein levels in hemodialysis patients. *Transplantation Proceedings*. 2004;36(1):38–40.

285 Goicoechea M, Caramelo C, Rodriguez P et al. Role of type of vascular access in erythropoietin and intravenous iron requirements in haemodialysis. *Nephrology Dialysis Transplantation*. 2001;16(11): 2188–2193.

286 Kato A, Odamaki M, Takita T et al. High blood soluble receptor p80 for tumour necrosis factor-alpha is associated with erythropoietin resistance in haemodialysis patients. *Nephrology Dialysis Transplantation*. 2001;16(9):1838–1844.

287 Anon. European best practice guidelines for the management of anemia in patients with chronic renal failure. *Nephrology Dialysis Transplantation*. 2004;19(Suppl 2):1.

288 Kharagjitsingh AV, Korevaar JC, Vandenbroucke JP et al. Incidence of recombinant erythropoietin (EPO) hyporesponse, EPO-associated antibodies, and pure red cell aplasia in dialysis patients. *Kidney International*. 2005;68(3):1215–1222.

289 Yaqoob M, Ahmad R, McClelland P et al. Resistance to recombinant human erythropoietin due to aluminium overload and its reversal by low dose desferrioxamine therapy. *Postgraduate Medical Journal*. 1993;69(808):124–128.

290 Verhelst D, Rossert J, Casadevall N et al. Treatment of erythropoietin-induced pure red cell aplasia: a retrospective study. *Lancet*. 2004;363(9423):1768–1771.

291 Cooper A, Mikhail A, Lethbridge MW et al. Pentoxifylline improves hemoglobin levels in patients with erythropoietin-resistant anemia in renal failure. *Journal of the American Society of Nephrology*. 2004;15(7):1877–1882.

292 PRCA Global Scientific Advisory Board. *PRCA*. Available from: www prcaforum com.

293 Roman RM, Lobo PI, Taylor RP et al. Prospective study of the immune effects of normalizing the hemoglobin concentration in hemodialysis patients who receive recombinant human erythropoietin. *Journal of the American Society of Nephrology*. 2004;15(5):1339–1346.

294 Jacobs C, Frei D, Perkins AC. Results of the European Survey on Anaemia Management 2003 (ESAM 2003): current status of anaemia management in dialysis patients, factors affecting epoetin dosage and changes in anaemia management over the last 5 years. *Nephrology Dialysis Transplantation*. 2005;20(Suppl 3):3–24.

295 Furuland H, Linde T, Ahlmen J et al. A randomized controlled trial of haemoglobin normalization with epoetin alfa in predialysis and dialysis patients. *Nephrology Dialysis Transplantation*. 2003;18(2):353–361.